SKIN OF COLOR SERIES

Dermatological

ATLAS *of* BLACK SKIN

COYLE CONNOLLY, D.O.

Assistant Clinical Professor of Dermatology,
Philadelphia College of Osteopathic Medicine, Philadelphia, PA, and
Lawrence Paolini & Coyle Connolly Dermatology and
Dermatologic Surgery, Cape May Court House, NJ.

JOSEPH BIKOWSKI, MD

Assistant Clinical Professor of Dermatology, University of
Pittsburgh, PA, and Sewickley Dermatological Associates, P.C.

merit
PUBLISHING
INTERNATIONAL

I

MERIT PUBLISHING INTERNATIONAL

NORTH AMERICAN ADDRESS:

8260 NW 49th Manor, Pine Grove
Coral Springs, Florida 33067
USA

EUROPEAN ADDRESS:

1st Floor, 35 Winchester Street
Basingstoke, Hampshire RG21 7EE,
Great Britain

ISBN: 1 873413 61 0

'To my mother and father in sunshine or in shadow'
Coyle

merit
PUBLISHING
INTERNATIONAL

SKIN OF COLOR SERIES

Dermatological

ATLAS *of* BLACK SKIN

COYLE CONNOLLY

JOSEPH BIKOWSKI

merit
PUBLISHING
INTERNATIONAL

CONTENTS

merit
PUBLISHING
INTERNATIONAL

INTRODUCTION

THE study of cutaneous diseases in black people is important for many reasons, not least because the black population represents a vital and expanding segment of the worldwide community. In the United States, for example, African Americans comprised approximately 12% of the entire population in 1990, and by the year 2050 this figure is expected to rise to 22%. Of the almost 39 million inhabitants of South Africa in 1991, 75.2% of the population were black Africans. The dermatological needs of this large ethnic group must be addressed on an international basis but unfortunately, a relative paucity of information exists regarding black skin and few textbooks have been exclusively devoted to this subject.

In the **DERMATOLOGICAL ATLAS OF BLACK SKIN** by Coyle Connolly and Joseph Bikowski, the authors address the clinical study of cutaneous diseases by examining high quality images accompanied by text. The information contained in the Atlas outlines the definition, etiology, clinical perspective, differential diagnosis, and treatment options for conditions affecting black skin. Physicians and medical students will be able to accurately recognize cutaneous diseases and learn how to effectively manage and treat them.

Covering 32 diseases, the authors examine clinical variations encountered in black patients and their distinctive color changes. Lesions appearing to be tan or red in Caucasians, for example, may look gray, purple or black in darker skinned individuals. Lichen planus, pityriasis rosea and psoriasis are just several examples of this unique color difference. Pigmentary alterations in the form of hypopigmentation and hyperpigmentation represent the most obvious, and often the most distressing, clinical changes in this ethnic group. Hypopigmented diseases include atopic dermatitis, idiopathic guttate hypomelanosis, pityriasis alba, post-inflammatory conditions, and vitiligo. Hyperpigmentation is seen in many post-inflammatory conditions and photosensitivity reactions.

Distinctive reaction patterns can be seen in black skin and hair. These patterns include follicular, ie. Fox-Fordyce Disease, papular, as in atopic dermatitis, annular, such as syphilis and sarcoidosis, and granulomatous responses. Generally, hair may be typed as straight, wavy, short, and helical or spiral (particularly in black people), which imparts a curl to the hair. These latter inherent hair properties make black hair more dry and brittle and, as a result, black people may need to use certain oily hair care products which sometimes lead to cutaneous disorders such as pomade acne. The curved hair and follicle play a central role in the etiology of several conditions manifesting as pseudofolliculitis barbae and acne keloidalis nuchae, which are more common in black people than Caucasians.

Black skin demonstrates normal variants which may be unknown to the less experienced physician. Concerned patients may seek medical attention for their benign condition and, if clinicians can recognize these variants, unnecessary treatments can be avoided. Education is required at all levels to ensure that clinicians are able to diagnose cutaneous diseases in black people. With the black population growing throughout the world, the clinical needs of this group are becoming more important.

The comprehensive coverage of cutaneous diseases in the **DERMATOLOGICAL ATLAS OF BLACK SKIN** will make an important contribution to the care and treatment of black people. It will provide physicians with a practical guide and an extremely useful reference source.

ACNE KELOIDALIS NUCHAE

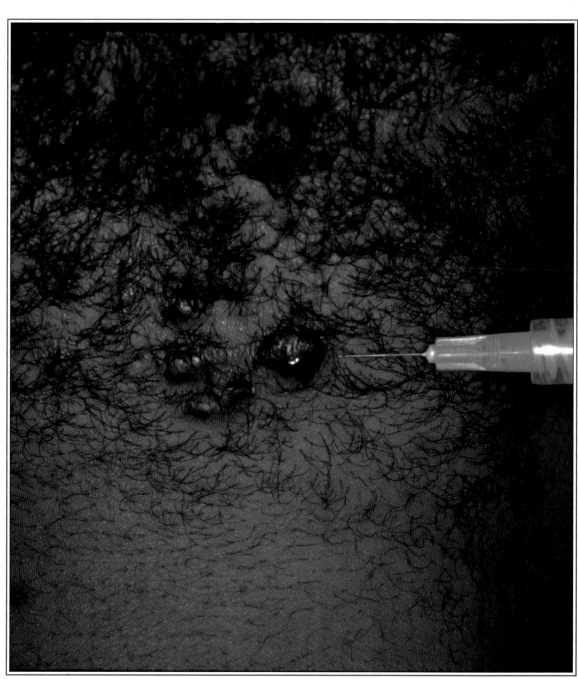

DEFINITION: Acne Keloidalis Nuchae is a chronic inflammatory disease involving the nape of the neck and occipital area.

ETIOLOGY: The precise etiology of Acne Keloidalis Nuchae is unknown. However, in black people both the hair shaft and follicle are curved and the curved hair may penetrate the dermis. The resultant embedded hairs may produce the follicular inflammation demonstrated on biopsy. Irritation from shirt collars may also play a causative role. Mostly black males are affected, although females who shave their necks too closely may develop lesions.

CLINICAL PERSPECTIVE: Folliculitis, ingrown hairs and keloids represent the constellation of findings seen in Acne Keloidalis Nuchae.

DIFFERENTIAL DIAGNOSIS: The finding of folliculitis, entrapped hair and keloids on the nape of the neck and occipital region, is quite distinctive.

TREATMENT OPTIONS: Treatments are directed towards each clinical component. Oral antibiotics, vitamin A, oral retinoids, benzoyl peroxide, chloramphenicol, and aluminum chloride solution are useful for the follicular component. Ingrown hairs are best treated by shaving avoidance (if possible) and mechanical extraction. Intralesional and topical corticosteroids, surgical excision, carbon dioxide laser, radiotherapy and cryosurgery may improve the keloidal component. It is also possible to freeze the papules with liquid nitrogen for 15-20 seconds and, after five minutes, intralesional corticosteroids may be injected into the lesion. The liquid nitrogen causes vasodilatation leading to edema which permits the corticosteroid to be injected with relative ease.

Atopic Dermatitis

TOP LEFT

Lichenification (an increase in the skin markings) is the hallmark of chronic atopic dermatitis. The thickened, hyperpigmented patches often occur on the flexural wrist, as seen in this 20-year-old atopic.

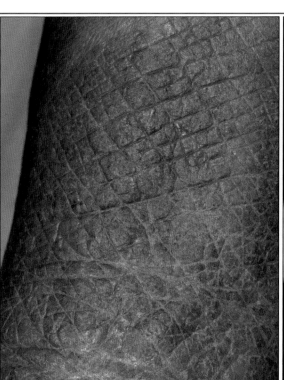

TOP RIGHT

A young atopic female is depicted scratching her arms. Young children with this condition often show involvement of the face and extensor arms and legs.

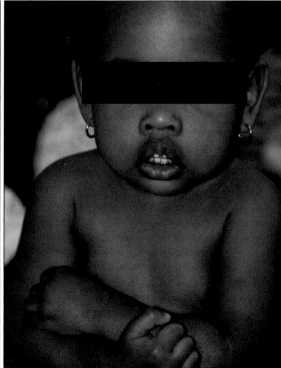

LOWER

Atopic dermatitis of the eyelids showing hyperpigmentation exacerbated by chronic rubbing.

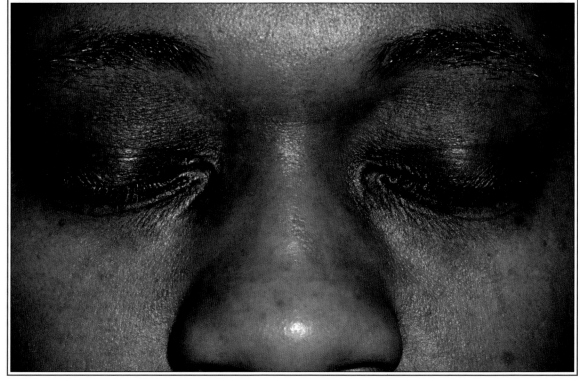

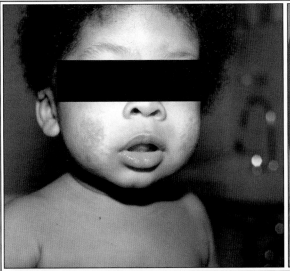

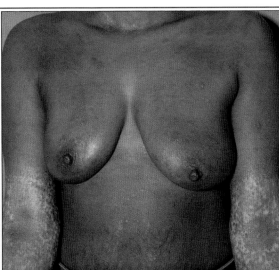

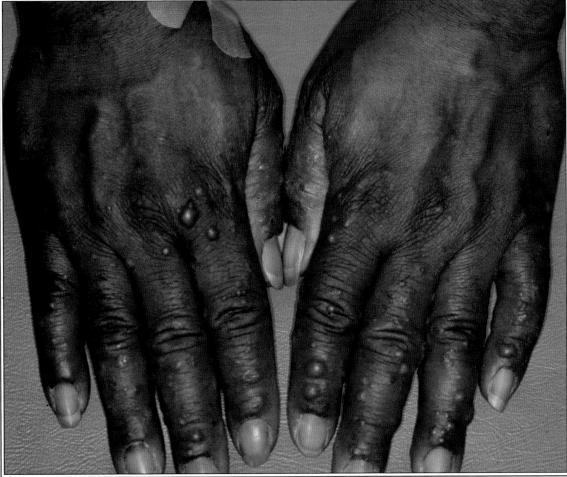

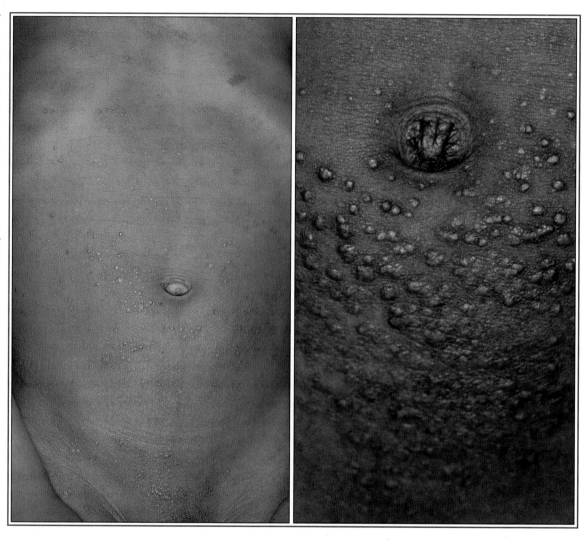

LEFT

Atopic Dermatitis in black people may have a distinctive follicular pattern. The otherwise healthy 6-year-old male pictured, reveals pruritic, brownish, discrete, 1-3 mm papules distributed on the abdomen and suprapubic region.

RIGHT

Hyperpigmented lichenified papules of the lower abdomen secondary to allergic contact dermatitis to nickel in a belt buckle. Papular atopic dermatitis may mimic this condition. A history of atopy and lichenified patches on the extremities help distinguish the two conditions.

DEFINITION: Atopic Dermatitis is a pruritic, acute, subacute, or chronic inflammation of the skin. A personal or family history of asthma, hay fever, eczema or hives is frequently found.

ETIOLOGY: Atopic Dermatitis is often referred to as the 'itch that rashes'. An itch is a stimulus that produces the urge to scratch. Dry skin, heat, humidity, perspiration, temperature change and anxiety may cause the itching sensation.

CLINICAL PERSPECTIVE: Atopic Dermatitis occurs in infant, childhood and adult phases. In ages two months to two years (infantile phase), the erythematous, scaling or weeping eruption is distributed primarily on the face and extensor surfaces of the extremities. In patients aged two years and older (childhood/adult phase), the disease is largely flexural. The antecubital fossae, popliteal fossae, flexor wrists and forearms, periorbital, perioral, hands, and feet may be affected.

A distinctive variation of Atopic Dermatitis, in the form of follicular papules, is more common among black children. Since follicular accentuation is not exclusive to this form of atopic dermatitis, a family history of atopy may suggest the correct diagnosis. Atopics with black skin also have a higher incidence of lichenified, hyperpigmented and hypopigmented lesions.

DIFFERENTIAL DIAGNOSIS: Contact Dermatitis (history of exposure to chemicals or medications); scabies (predilection for finger web spaces, waist, axillae, close contacts often with similar eruption, worse at night, 2-4 mm linear 'burrows'); Wiskott-Aldrich syndrome (rare immunodeficiency, male infants affected, eczematous dermatitis, recurrent bacterial infections).

ASSOCIATIONS: Xerosis, ichthyosis vulgaris, keratosis pilaris, pityriasis alba, atopic pleats (Dennie-Morgan folds), white dermatographism and anterior subcapsular cataracts may accompany atopic dermatitis.

TREATMENT OPTIONS: Antihistamines, topical tars, moisturizers and corticosteroids are the mainstays of therapy. Caution must be used when treating with high potency topical corticosteroids for extended periods of time, due to the increased risk of steroid-induced hypopigmentation in black people.

DERMATOSIS PAPULOSA NIGRA

TOP

The benign condition of dermatosis papulosa nigra can be seen on the cheeks and temple of this 40-year-old female.

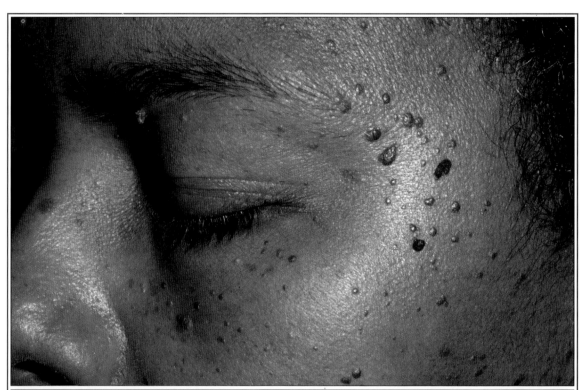

LOWER

A 41-year-old female complained of 'flesh moles' on her cheeks. These small dark brown papules on the malar region are typical of dermatosis papulosa nigra.

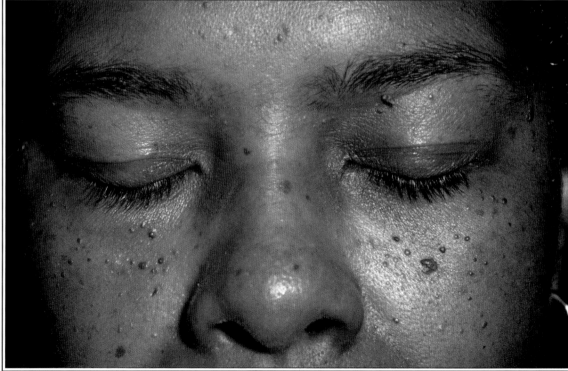

DEFINITION: Dermatosis Papulosa Nigra consists of dark brown papules, 1-5 mm, usually located on the malar region.

ETIOLOGY: Between 35 and 77% of black patients may be affected. Over 50% of patients have a family history of similar lesions and there appears to be a female predilection with a peak incidence during the sixth decade. Dermatosis Papulosa Nigra has been reported in patients as young as three years of age. The lesions are histologically indistinguishable from seborrheic keratoses.

CLINICAL PERSPECTIVE: These benign, brown to black papules may involve the neck, trunk and shoulders in addition to the typical malar distribution.

DIFFERENTIAL DIAGNOSIS: Nevi and fibroepithelial polyps can mimic Dermatosis Papulosa Nigra. The aforementioned conditions are not confined to the malar area.

TREATMENT OPTIONS: Patients may desire cosmetic treatment for these 'flesh moles', as they are sometimes referred to by patients. Scissor excision, electrodessication and liquid nitrogen are all useful treatments. Scissor excision is preferred, since overaggressive electrodessication or prolonged liquid nitrogen application may lead to scarring or post-inflammatory hypopigmentation.

DISSECTING CELLULITIS OF THE SCALP

TOP

The occipital scalp of a 32-year-old pharmacist with multiple, painful, boggy nodules leading to the condition termed dissecting cellulitis of the scalp. Patchy alopecia is also observed.

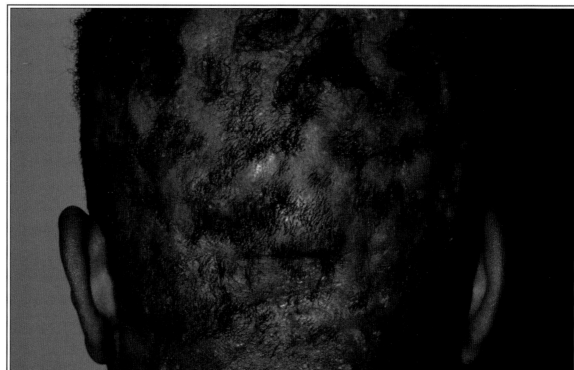

LOWER

A round, elevated inflamed plaque studded with pustules on the right scalp of a 22-year-old male with kerion formation. Culture of the area showed co-infection with Staphylococcus aureus. The lesion cleared after a one month course of an oral antifungal and oral antibiotic.

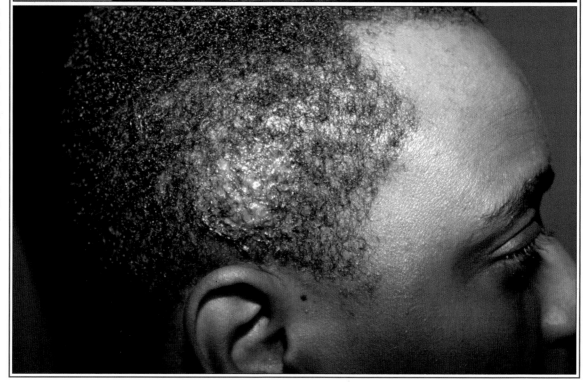

DEFINITION: Dissecting Cellulitis of the Scalp *(perifolliculitis capitis abscedens et suffodiens)* is a chronic suppurative condition seen mostly in young black males.

ETIOLOGY: The exact cause of Dissecting Cellulitis is unknown but follicular occlusion and a granulomatous reaction to keratin may be implicated. This disease is almost unique to black people.

CLINICAL PERSPECTIVE:

The painful nodules and abscesses are typically located on the vertex and occiput. Sinus tract formation is a common feature and infectious organisms including Staphylococcus aureus and pseudomonas have been isolated from the draining sinuses. Scarring alopecia and keloid formation represent late sequelae.

ASSOCIATIONS: When Dissecting Cellulitis of the Scalp occurs in conjunction with acne conglobata and hidradenitis suppurativa, the follicular occlusion triad is formed.

DIFFERENTIAL DIAGNOSIS: Kerions associated with tinea infection evolve over a shorter period of time than Dissecting Cellulitis of the Scalp. A fungal culture is often helpful.

TREATMENT OPTIONS: Treatments should target the inflammatory component and stabilize the follicular lining. An anti-inflammatory effect is provided by corticosteroids, dapsone, and zinc, and retinoic acid appears to exert a beneficial effect on follicular keratinization. Incision and drainage, surgical excision and X-ray therapy may sometimes be required and long-term oral and topical antibiotics are usually necessary.

Drug-induced Photosensitivity Reaction

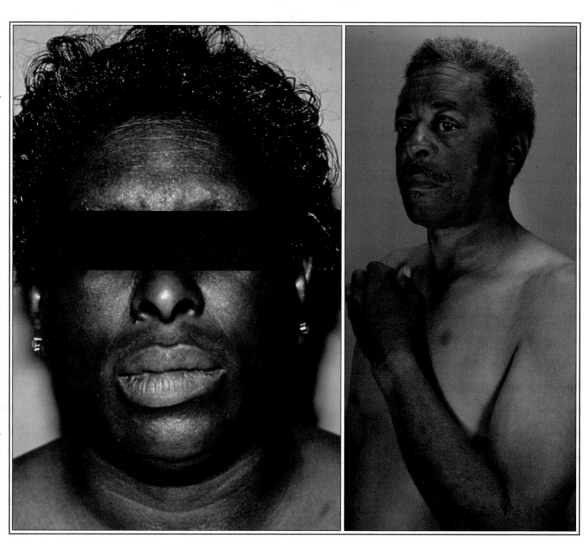

LEFT
Photosensitivity reaction secondary to soap in a 38-year-old female. Note the hyperpigmentation of the forehead, cheeks, upper lip, and neck. The sun protected areas of the upper philtrum and submental region were spared in this light sensitive dermatosis.

RIGHT
This 53-year-old male presented with a one year history of pruritic, scaling, hyperpigmented patches confined to the sun exposed areas of the face, 'v' of the neck and extensor forearms. No skin changes were found in the area protected by his watch. Ingestion of a thiazide diuretic caused this photoallergic eruption.

DEFINITION: Photosensitivity reactions occur when an external or internally ingested substance exposed to ultraviolet light produces an abnormal skin response.

ETIOLOGY: Photosensitivity reactions are classified into photoallergic and phototoxic forms. Photoallergic reactions are cell mediated while phototoxic reactions are non-immunologic. Drugs associated with photoallergic and phototoxic dermatoses are listed in Table 1.

CLINICAL PERSPECTIVE: Drug Induced Photosensitivity Reactions produce erythema on sun exposed areas. Sites of predilection include the forehead, nose, malar region, neck, 'V' of the chest, extensor forearms and dorsal hands. Areas covered by hair, upper eyelids, melolabial folds, upper cutaneous lip, and the submental region are characteristically spared. In females, the legs are often involved. Photoallergic eruptions are pruritic, eczematous or vesicular and are clinically similar to allergic contact dermatitis. Phototoxic eruptions are erythematous, edematous and resemble an irritant contact dermatitis. Patients with the aforementioned condition will often complain of a burning sensation.

The erythema associated with photosensitivity reactions is more difficult to recognize in black people due to 'masking' by the darker skin pigment. Black skin is less susceptible to these reactions than Caucasian skin. Phototoxic reactions are rare in very dark skinned black people and photoallergic reactions are the most severe in the more deeply pigmented patients.

DIFFERENTIAL DIAGNOSIS: Photoallergic reactions may resemble airborne allergic contact dermatitis, atopic dermatitis and polymorphous light eruption. Phototoxic reactions may cause confusion with severe sunburn, lupus erythematosus and the porphyrias. Laboratory tests (ANA, porphyrin levels), photopatch testing (for photoallergic reactions), and patient history will help the physician reach the correct diagnosis.

TREATMENT OPTIONS: The offending internal or external drug should be identified and removed. Sunscreens, topical or oral corticosteroids and antihistamines are beneficial.

FOX-FORDYCE DISEASE

Fox-Fordyce disease. Multiple, discrete, firm papules involving the axilla and breast of a 27-year-old female.

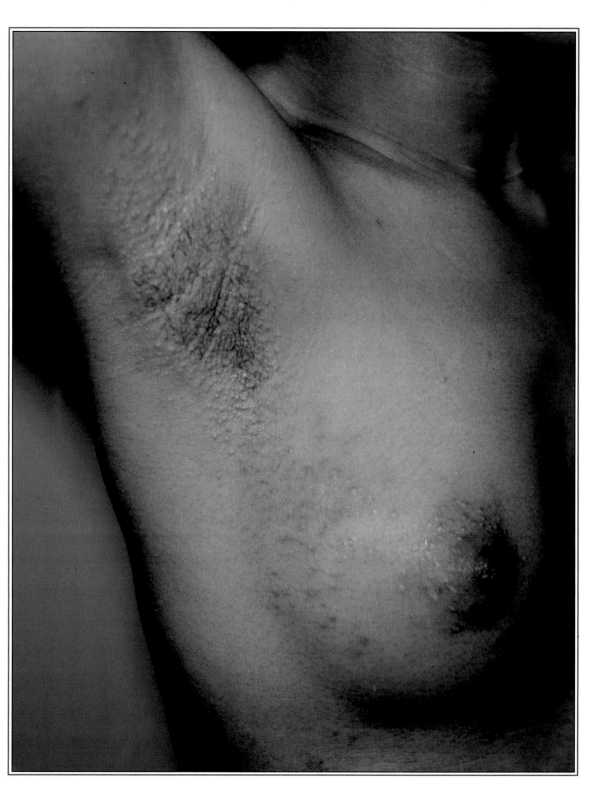

DEFINITION: Fox-Fordyce Disease, or apocrine miliaria, is a chronic and pruritic disorder due to apocrine duct obstruction.

ETIOLOGY: The cause is unknown. Microscopic examination reveals a keratotic plug blocking the ostium of the apocrine duct. Black females are primarily affected, although males, children and identical twins may present with this disease.

CLINICAL PERSPECTIVE: Tan to brown, discrete, follicular papules are found in the axillae. Less frequently, the areolae or anogenital areas may be involved.

DIFFERENTIAL DIAGNOSIS: Montgomery's tubercles, which become prominent during pregnancy, may simulate Fox-Fordyce Disease.

TREATMENT OPTIONS: A protracted course may be anticipated and medical treatments are often unsatisfactory. Tretinoin cream, clindamycin solution, intralesional corticosteroids, isotretinoin, and ultraviolet light have all been attempted with varying success. Electrodessication and surgical excision may be successful in resistant cases. Fox-Fordyce Disease usually improves with pregnancy and may respond to oral contraceptives, suggesting a hormonal influence.

FUTCHER'S LINES

A subtle streak of pigmentary demarcation, or Futcher's line, is evident on the upper arm of this 26-year-old secretary. The longitudinal line divides the darker lateral portion from the lighter medial portion.

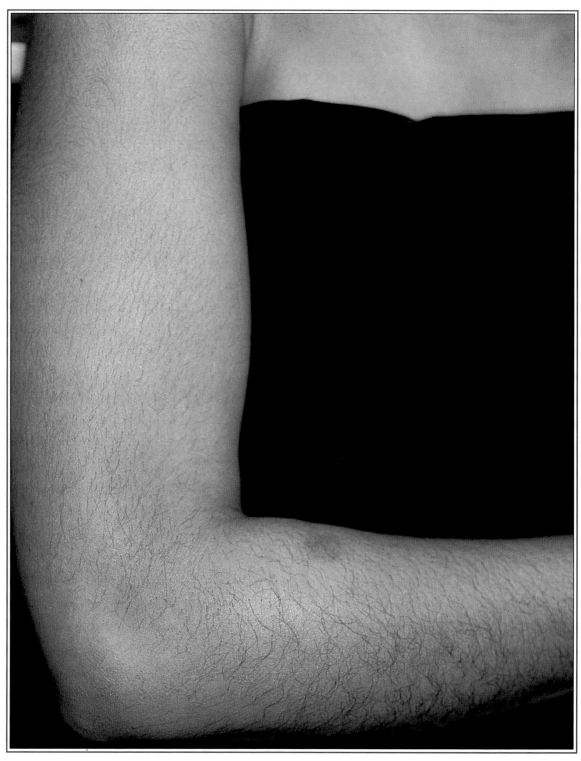

DEFINITION: Futcher's [60] or Voigt's lines are sharp, bilateral, pigmentary demarcation lines usually located on the arms and legs. This condition represents a normal variant in black people.

ETIOLOGY: Futcher's lines correspond to the underlying spinal nerves innervating a dermatome. An incidence of 25% has been reported in heavily pigmented black persons. James[62], et al. found that 79% of black females had at least one type of line. Some of the black women studied first noticed the Futcher's lines during pregnancy and in the majority of cases, pigmentation lines are present at birth. Interestingly, biopsy reveals that the hyperpigmentation is not due to an increase in melanin.

CLINICAL PERSPECTIVE: Futcher's lines separate the darker anterolateral region from the lighter anteromedial region.

DIFFERENTIAL DIAGNOSIS: The finding of symmetrical, linear hyperpigmented streaks is quite distinctive.

TREATMENT OPTIONS: Reassurance is all that is required for this benign condition.

GINGIVAL
HYPERPIGMENTATION

Gingival hyper-pigmentation, a normal variant in black people, is demonstrated in this 19-year-old male. One should inquire about ingested medications (i.e., antimalarials) which may mimic this benign condition.

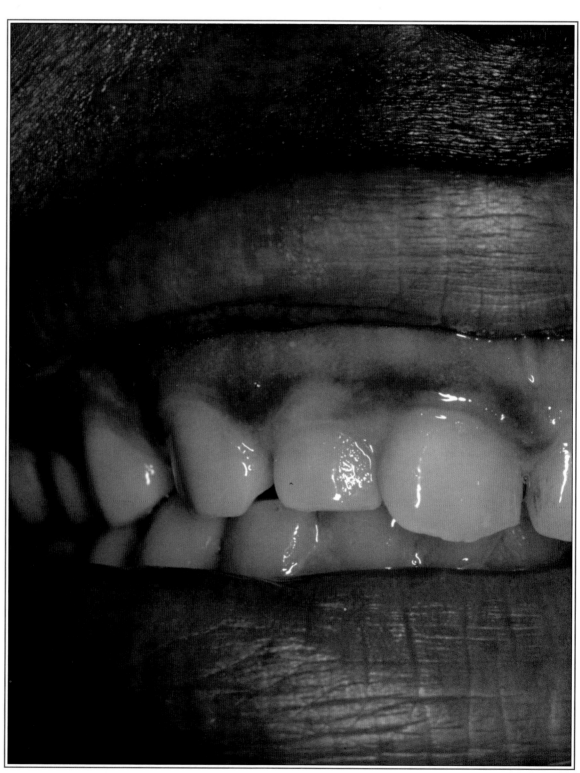

DEFINITION: The gingival mucosa may demonstrate a light brown to dark brown, symmetrical discoloration in black people.

ETIOLOGY: Gingival Hyperpigmentation represents a normal variant among black people. The incidence of oral pigmentation is greater in darkly pigmented black skin. However, the degree of patient skin pigmentation does not correlate with the degree of oral pigmentation. There are many deeply pigmented individuals with no signs of this condition.

CLINICAL PERSPECTIVE: Most often, the anterior gingiva are involved. The buccal mucosa, hard palate and tongue (especially the anterior papillae), are affected to a lesser degree.

DIFFERENTIAL DIAGNOSIS: Certain drugs (antimalarials, phenothiazine) and heavy metals may cause oral pigmentation. This underscores the need for a careful drug ingestion history. Addison's disease, Peutz-Jegher's syndrome and hemochromatosis must also be considered in the differential diagnosis.

TREATMENT OPTIONS: Intervention is not necessary due to the benign nature of this condition.

IDIOPATHIC GUTTATE
HYPOMELANOSIS

Idiopathic guttate hypomelanosis: discrete, innumerable, white, irregularly bordered 2-4 mm macules of the lower leg in a 50-year-old female. These lesions, unlike vitiligo, are hypopigmented rather than depigmented.

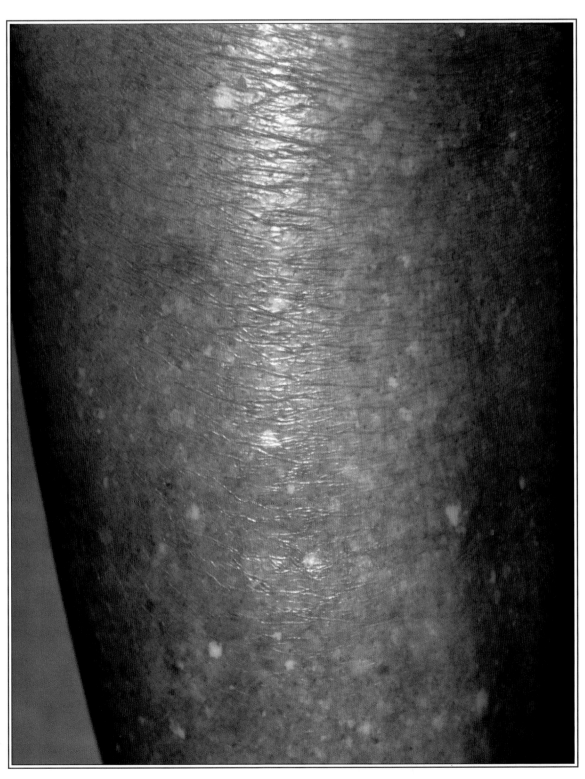

DEFINITION: Idiopathic Guttate Hypomelanosis, or Disseminate Lenticular Leucoderma, comprises small, white, irregularly shaped macules occurring mostly on the anterior lower legs.

ETIOLOGY: Actinic damage has been proposed as a cause of Idiopathic Guttate Hypomelanosis in Caucasians. The etiology is poorly understood in black people. Histologically, a decrease in the number of melanocytes is found and women, especially those over 40 years of age, represent the majority of cases.

CLINICAL PERSPECTIVE: The discrete, hypopigmented macules range in size from 2-6 mm and possess an irregular border. The disease is more noticeable in black people than Caucasians, and may involve the trunk as well as legs.

DIFFERENTIAL DIAGNOSIS: Unlike Idiopathic Guttate Hypomelanosis, vitiligo tends to be periorificial and not confined to the lower legs.

TREATMENT OPTIONS: Triamcinilone acetonide may be injected intralesionally if the lesions are cosmetically objectionable. Usually, no treatment is required.

KELOIDS

A 35-year-old male with many brown, firm nodules of the chest and abdomen. These keloids serve as a painful reminder of the varicella infection he had as a child.

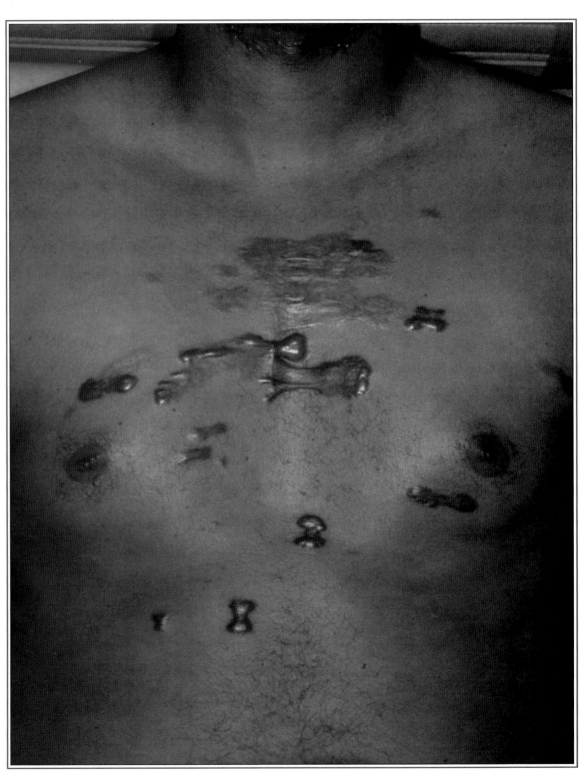

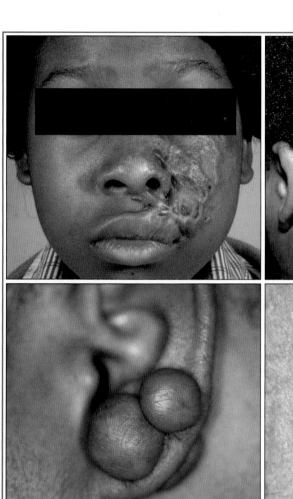

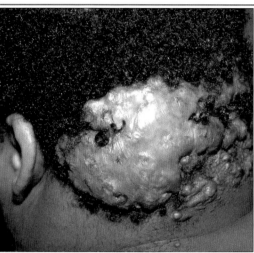

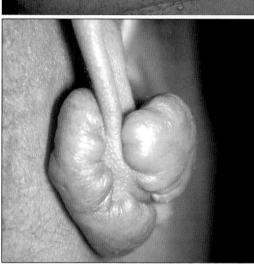

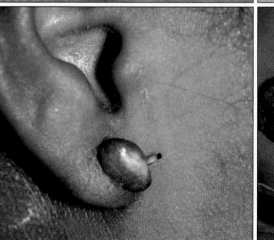

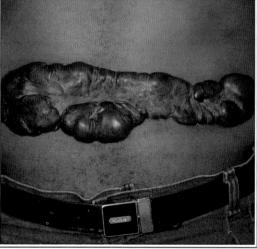

TOP LEFT

This 13-year-old female developed disfiguring facial keloids following a herpes zoster infection.

TOP RIGHT

A 22-year-old farmer with a keloidal mass involving the occipital region presents a therapeutic challenge. Ultimately, surgery with scalp reduction was required.

MIDDLE LEFT

A 23- year-old female with large, protuberant, flesh colored nodules of the anterior and posterior earlobe. Keloids are not uncommonly found in black people following ear piercing.

MIDDLE RIGHT

This 19-year-old female has large, pedunculated nodular keloids of the anterior and posterior ear lobe.

LOWER LEFT

Surgical excision may be the only option in patients such as this 22-year-old female who developed a 1.5 cm keloid on the anterior ear lobe following ear piercing.

LOWER RIGHT

An accidental laceration from barbed wire lead to this massive, dark brown, abdominal keloid in a 19-year-old male. The keloid recurred three times after surgical correction was attempted. Such recurrences are common in surgically treated keloids.

TOP LEFT
This unfortunate 30-year-old burn victim developed an extensive linear keloid on the lateral neck.

TOP MIDDLE
These 1-4 cm flesh colored nodules on the dorsal feet of this 22-year-old surfer from California represent hyperplastic granulomas or surfer's nodules. Repeated trauma from paddling the boards in the kneeling position is causative.

TOP RIGHT
Close up view of surfer's nodules which may be mistaken for keloids.

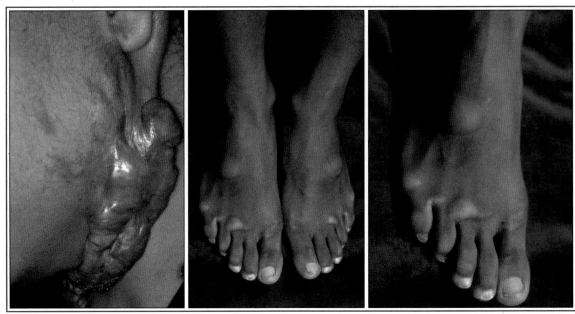

DEFINITION: Keloids are proliferative growths of dermal collagen.

ETIOLOGY: Keloids often occur in response to trauma and may be induced by abrasions, surgical procedures, ear piercing, burns, insect bites, and acne. Keloid formation can also occur following infection. In addition, an idiopathic type has been reported. Black people are two to nineteen times more likely to develop Keloids than their Caucasian counterparts.

Collagen deposition (type I and type VI) and transforming growth factor beta (TGFß) are increased. TGFß, a collagenase inhibitor, activates collagen production, and currently, investigators are examining the effectiveness of TGFß antagonists for the treatment of Keloids.

CLINICAL PERSPECTIVE: These firm, flesh colored nodules are often asymptomatic, although pruritis and tenderness may be encountered. Unfortunately, Keloids may reach considerable sizes and cause disfigurement. Sites of predilection include the earlobes, shoulders and upper thorax.

DIFFERENTIAL DIAGNOSIS: Unlike hypertrophic scars, Keloids extend beyond the original injury site in a claw-like manner. The word Keloid is derived from the Greek word *chele*, meaning 'crab claw'.

TREATMENT OPTIONS: Both non-surgical and surgical techniques have been utilized to treat Keloids. Non-surgical modalities include corticosteroids, tretinoin, pressure garments, and pressure earrings. Liquid nitrogen can be used to soften Keloids prior to corticosteroid injections. Liquid nitrogen is also capable of treating Keloids directly and the freeze cycle should last approximately 30 seconds. Silicone gel sheeting has recently gained popularity as a treatment. Some investigators begin silicone dressings immediately after wound healing in Keloid formers. A silicone occlusive sheet worn daily for up to nine months was shown to improve Keloids in 88% of treated subjects. Investigators speculate that the silicone may create an electrical field which inhibits scar tissue formation. Corticosteroid tape occlusion is useful in early Keloids. Minoxidil lotion inhibits fibroblast activity in vitro and may prove beneficial, and Interferon gamma and other TGFß antagonists hold future promise.

Surgical excision may be used alone or in combination with intralesional corticosteroids, methotrexate and radiation. Surgery, in conjunction with radiation, offers the lowest recurrence rate. Kantor [90], et al. successfully treated Keloids with a carbon dioxide laser and pulsed dye lasers may be effective for erythematous Keloids.

Prevention is thought to be the most important factor in reducing the likelihood of Keloid formation. All unnecessary cosmetic surgery should be avoided in patients with a history of Keloids. Careful surgical planning will minimize Keloid development and placing incisions along skin tension lines, avoiding undue skin tension and proper suturing techniques are vital. Despite prevention and proper treatment, Keloids may recur. Recurrence rates are highest in patients with a history of wound site infection or a positive family history.

LEUKOEDEMA

A 32-year-old non-smoker presented with white, non-scaling patches of the oral cavity. The correct diagnosis is leukoedema.

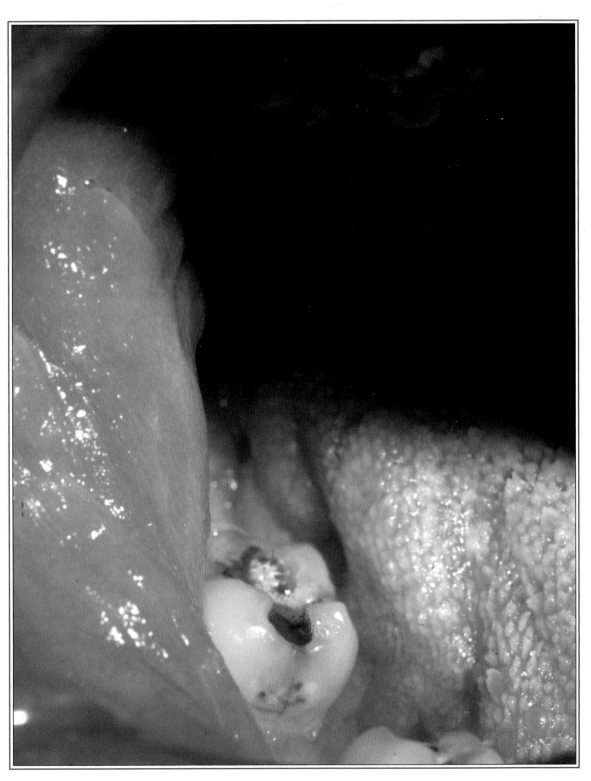

DEFINITION: Oral leukoedema is a benign condition affecting up to 90% of black people.

ETIOLOGY: Cigarette smoking and poor oral hygiene may be causative in some cases. Microscopic examination reveals epidermal edema. There is no sex predilection.

CLINICAL PERSPECTIVE: Leukoedema presents as white, non-scaling patches located on the buccal mucosa.

DIFFERENTIAL DIAGNOSIS: Leukoplakia may develop in leukoedematous lesions and close oral surveillance is warranted. Oral lichen planus may present on the buccal mucosa as a reticulated white patch. A search for the typical violaceous papules of lichen planus in other locations should be undertaken.

TREATMENT OPTIONS: Treatment is not necessary for this benign, normal variant.

LICHEN NITIDUS

TOP

An example of lichen nitidus involving the penile shaft of a 27-year-old male. These discrete and grouped, shiny papules may occasionally be mistaken for genital warts. However, the uniform size and distribution of lesions in lichen nitidus will lead to the correct diagnosis.

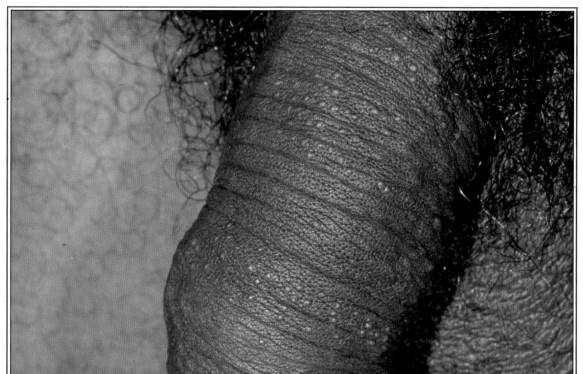

LOWER

Numerous, 1-2 mm tan papules on the corona caused great alarm in this 17-year-old black male. These benign, pearly, penile papules represent angiofibromas histologically. The characteristic size and location on the corona or coronal sulcus distinguish this condition from condyloma acuminata and lichen nitidus.

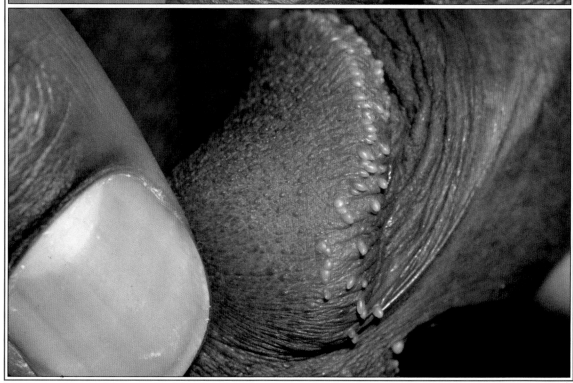

DEFINITION: Lichen Nitidus consists of asymptomatic, shiny, pinpoint papules found on the trunk, wrists and genitalia.

ETIOLOGY: The exact cause of Lichen Nitidus is unknown but hormonal factors may play a role. While there is no racial predilection, the lesions are more apparent in black skin. Lichen Nitidus is also more common in children, especially black males.

CLINICAL PERSPECTIVE: The non-pruritic, shiny 1-2 mm papules are quite striking in black patients. Sites of predilection include the chest, abdomen, arms, penis and buttocks. Nail changes associated with Lichen Nitidus include linear striations, ridging and irregular pitting.

ASSOCIATIONS: Lichen Nitidus may co-exist with lichen planus in as many as 25-30% of cases. A rare association with Crohn's disease has been described.

DIFFERENTIAL DIAGNOSIS: The differential diagnosis includes lichen planus (violaceous, predilection for wrists, ankles); micropapular sarcoidosis (non-caseating granulomas on biopsy); pearly penile papules (localized to coronal sulcus); keratosis pilaris (posterior arms), and lichen scrofulosorum (positive tuberculin reaction).

TREATMENT OPTIONS: Treatment is usually not required since most cases of Lichen Nitidus will resolve spontaneously. Topical corticosteroids and PUVA (psoralen and ultraviolet A light) therapy have helped older patients with diffuse involvement. More recently, oral astemizole has been successful. A case of recurrent generalized Lichen Nitidus associated with amenorrhea improved after estrogen and progesterone treatment. This suggests that hormonal factors may play a role in this disease.

LICHEN PLANUS

LEFT

Lichen planus often occurs on the glans penis. This 20-year-old incorrectly believed he had contracted a venereal disease. The deeply violaceous pruritic papules responded well to topical corticosteroids.

RIGHT

A 26-year-old female with striking gray-violaceous, annular, slightly raised plaques of the upper arm. This represents a case of annular lichen planus.

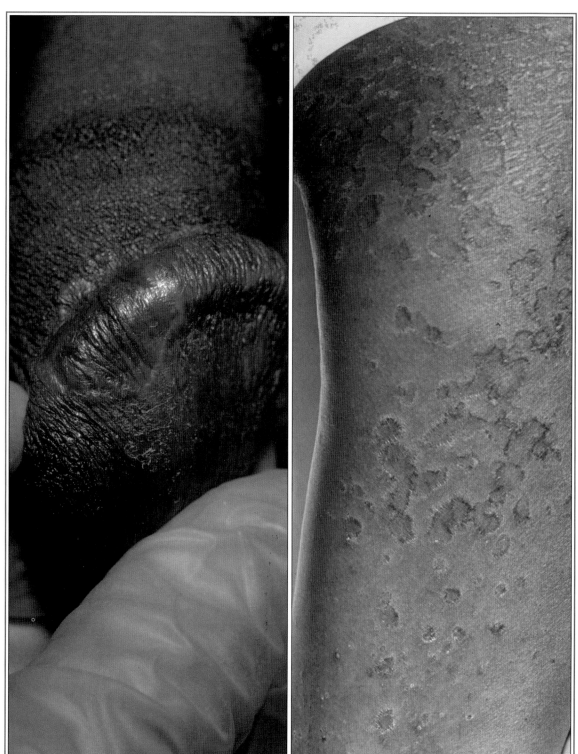

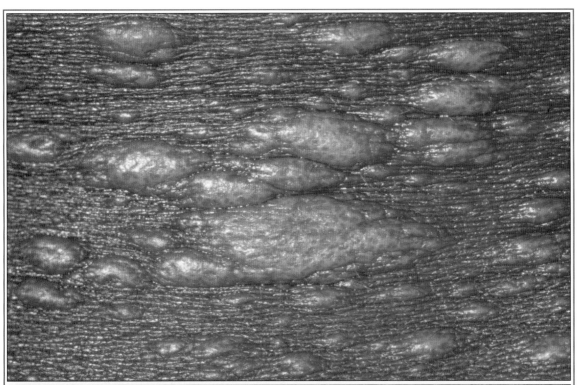

The typical flat-topped polygonal pruritic papules of lichen planus on the lower posterior thorax of an 18-year-old female student. Note the deep purple-gray color so characteristic in black people with this disease.

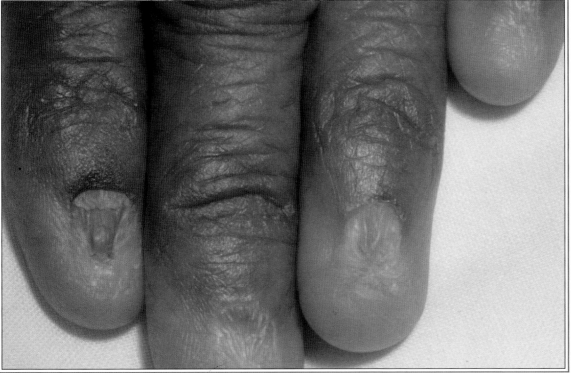

LOWER

A 70-year-old retired railroad engineer with nail destruction and pterygium formation of the hand. Lichen planus of the nails occurs in about ten percent of cases.

LICHEN PLANUS

(CONTINUED)

LEFT

The anterior tibial region of a 42-year-old female with hypertrophic lichen planus. These lesions are often verrucous with fine white adherent scale typically involving the lower extremities.

RIGHT

Another example of the hypertrophic form of Lichen Planus occuring on the anterior lower leg of a young female. The deeply purple-gray color is striking in black people with this disease.

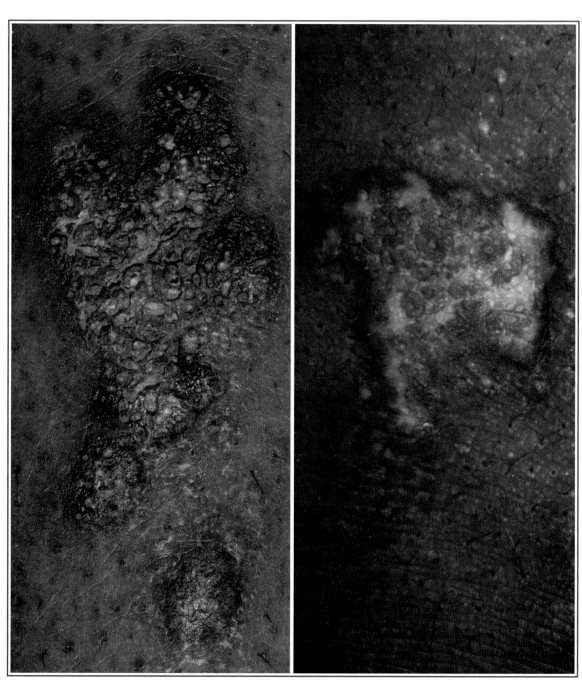

DEFINITION: This papulosquamous disease occurs mostly on the flexor wrists, ankles and mucous membranes.

ETIOLOGY: Lichen Planus may be precipitated by drugs (ACE inhibitors, antimalarials, diuretics) and contact with certain chemicals such as color film developer. A cell-mediated cytotoxic immune reaction may play a role.

CLINICAL PERSPECTIVE: The violaceous, scaling, flat-topped polygonal papules of Lichen Planus are often pruritic. Annular, linear, hypertrophic, follicular, vesicular, ulcerative, atrophic, actinic, and erythematous forms exist. Nail involvement occurs in 10% of patients and longitudinal grooving, ridging and pterygium formation represent potential nail changes.

In black people, the lesions tend to be deep purple or gray in color. A hypertrophic form is not uncommonly found. In Caucasians, 30-70% will have oral involvement. In contrast, black persons rarely manifest oral Lichen Planus. Finally, post-inflammatory hyperpigmentation may cause concern in darker skinned individuals.

DIFFERENTIAL DIAGNOSIS: Other papulosquamous diseases should be considered when entertaining a diagnosis of Lichen Planus. Psoriasis has a predilection for the scalp, elbows and knees. The scale in psoriasis is thick and micaceous compared to the more delicate, reticulate scale (Wickham's striae) found in Lichen Planus. The 'red brick' color of psoriatic lesions varies from the violaceous color of lichen planus. This color distinction is, of course, more subtle in black patients.

TREATMENT OPTIONS: The disease is usually self-limited and will often resolve within one to two years. Topical corticosteroids, with or without occlusion, and, rarely, short courses of oral corticosteroids may be necessary. Intralesional corticosteroids may be injected into hypertrophic lesions. Photochemotherapy, retinoids or cyclosporines may be required for severe or widespread disease. Oral antifungals may be attempted in difficult cases.

MIDLINE
HYPOPIGMENTATION

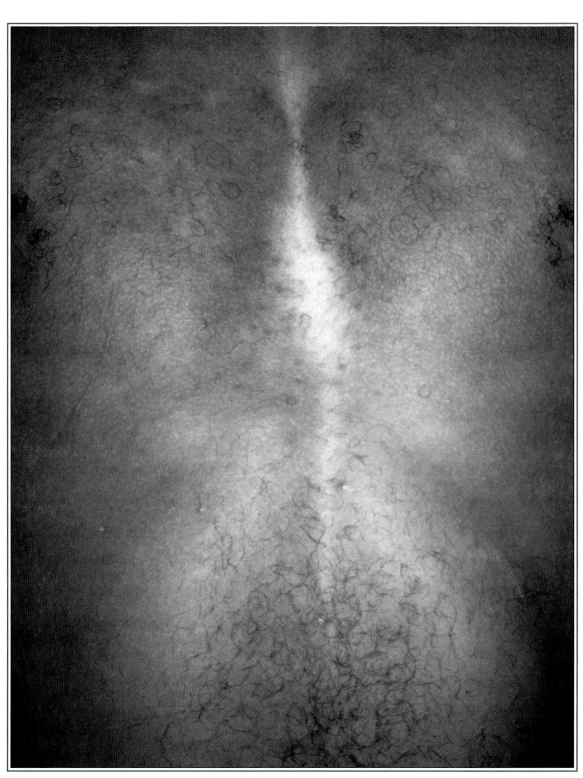

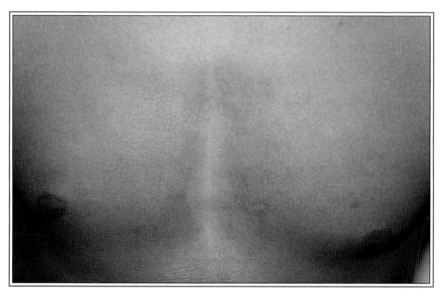

DEFINITION: Midline Hypopigmentation is seen as a linear band overlying the sternum.

ETIOLOGY: The precise etiology is unknown but this band may be inherited in an autosomal dominant pattern. The incidence of Midline Hypopigmentation in black people is reported to be approximately 30-40%. Black males are primarily affected and the hypopigmentation becomes less noticeable with advancing age.

CLINICAL PERSPECTIVE: This hypopigmented line may extend inferiorly from the sternum to involve the linea alba, or superiorly to involve the infraclavicular region.

DIFFERENTIAL DIAGNOSIS: Vitiligo is often symmetrically distributed with a predilection for the hands, feet and periorificial areas. Post-inflammatory hypopigmentation can be ruled out through a detailed history.

TREATMENT OPTIONS: Medical intervention is not required for this normal variant.

Mongolian Spot

A blue-gray patch on the posterior thorax represents a mongolian spot. The mother of this 2-year-old was concerned for her child's health. She was reassured that the benign lesions would fade and disappear with time.

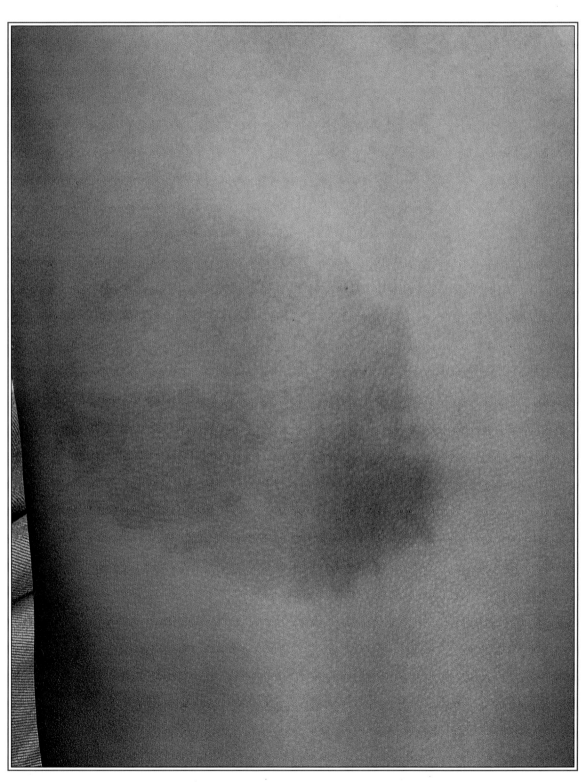

DEFINITION: The Mongolian Spot is a congenital blue-gray patch usually located lumbosacrally.

ETIOLOGY: The pigmentation is due to melanocytes in the dermis, hence the synonym, 'dermal melanocytosis'. The lesions eventually disappear by the age of six or seven and rarely persist into adulthood.

Although found mostly in Asians, between 40-90% of black neonates may show involvement. Only 10% of Caucasians exhibit Mongolian Spots.

CLINICAL PERSPECTIVE: The bluish gray patches are devoid of scale and often singular. Multiple lesions may be located in areas other than the lumbosacral region.

ASSOCIATIONS: The phakomatosis pigmentovascularis type IVa comprises a Mongolian spot, nevus spilus and nevus flammeus.

DIFFERENTIAL DIAGNOSIS: It is important to educate concerned family members and physicians that this is not a form of child abuse.

TREATMENT OPTIONS: The treatment is reassurance, since most lesions disappear with time.

NAIL PIGMENTATION

TOP LEFT

Multiple melanocytic striae of the nails in a 40-year-old male. This condition represents a normal variant.

TOP RIGHT

This pigmented compound nevus in a young adult male was biopsied to rule out subungual melanoma.

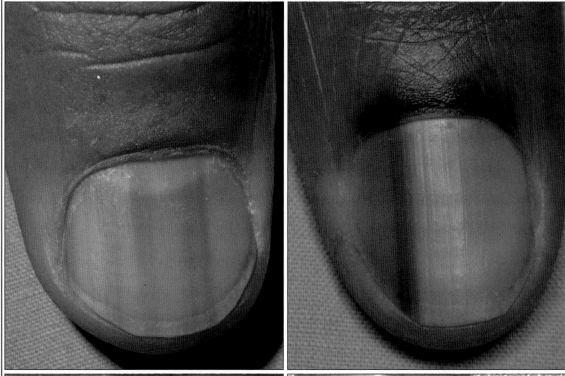

LOWER LEFT

Striking, linear, dark brown-black streak on the index finger of a female with benign nail pigmentation.

LOWER RIGHT

Linear hyperpigmented nail streaks on the bilateral thumbs of a 42-year-old female secondary to hydroxyurea. A careful drug history is vital in differentiating pigmented nail lesions.

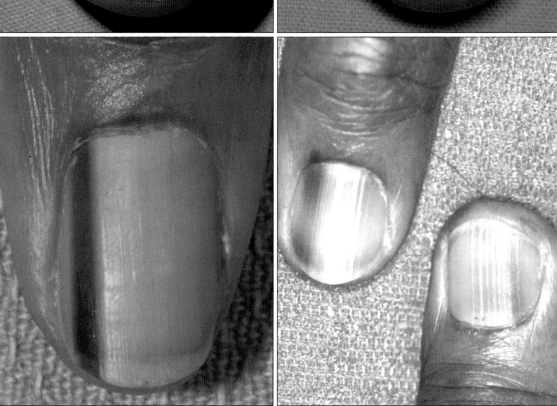

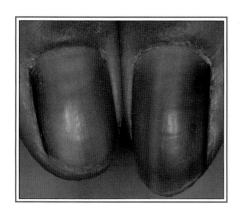

Hyperpigmentation of the nails in a patient taking Zidovudine. A careful drug history distinguishes this condition from nail pigmentation commonly found in black patients.

DEFINITION: Linear hyperpigmented nail streaks represent a normal variant in over 50% of black people.

ETIOLOGY: Trauma, or perhaps ultraviolet light, may play a role in the etiology of this disorder, where melanin is deposited in the nail plate and matrix. A positive correlation between increasing age and the frequency and intensity of the pigmentation exists.

CLINICAL PERSPECTIVE: The nails on the thumb and index finger are mostly affected. These brown colored bands are often bilaterally distributed. Occasionally, a diffuse pigmentation of the nails occurs instead of the longitudinal bands.

DIFFERENTIAL DIAGNOSIS: Drugs such as antimalarials, bleomycin, doxorubicin, and zidovudine may cause nail pigmentation. Systemic diseases such as Addison's disease and Peutz Jegher's disease must be considered in the differential diagnosis. Radiation has been reported as a cause of melanonychia. Melanoma is usually a single, unilateral lesion. Any irregular nail pigment or history of a changing lesion warrants a biopsy since as many as 20% of melanomas in black people are found in the nails. Junctional nevi may also be confused with the normal variant.

TREATMENT OPTIONS: Patient reassurance is all that is needed.

TOP

A 19-year-old female demonstrates a bluish-gray patch of the malar cheek which proved to be Nevus of Ota. Note the similar bluish pigmentation of the sclera, a frequently involved site in this disease. When ocular involvement occurs, a ophthalmologic examination is necessary to detect any associated glaucoma or melanoma.

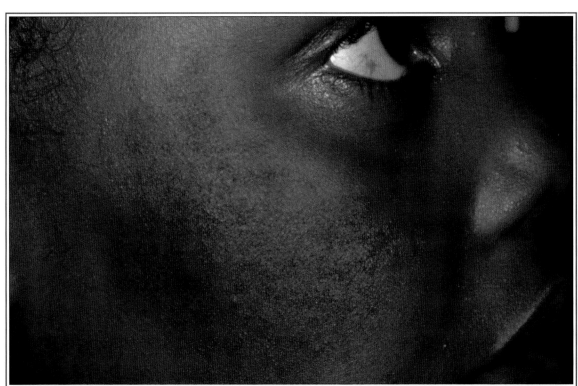

LOWER

This 24-year-old female was concerned about the cosmetic appearance of her Nevus of Ota which involved the periocular region and cheek. The pigmentation in this patient took on a brownish gray hue rather than the more common bluish-gray coloration. Scleral involvement was absent.

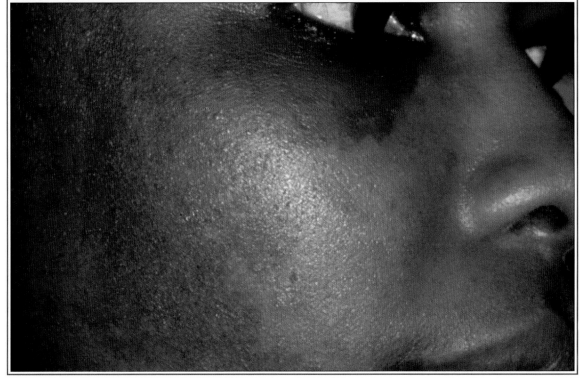

DEFINITION: Nevus of Ota (oculodermal melanocytosis) is a benign, blue-gray patch involving the skin innervated by cranial nerve V.

ETIOLOGY: The condition is felt to be due to an arrest in migration of melanocytes from the neural crest to the epidermis. Most cases are congenital, although many cases arise during childhood or puberty. An acquired lesion was reported in an 81-year-old adult. Lesions tend to persist into adulthood and there is a female preponderance. The nevus of Ota is most common among Asians, although black people are affected more often than Caucasians.

CLINICAL PERSPECTIVE: A diffuse blue-gray pigmentation is found on the eyelids, conjunctiva, sclera, cheeks, forehead and ears. Ocular pigmentation occurs in roughly 66% of patients. Glaucoma, conjunctival melanoma and meningeal melanoma have been documented in patients with the Nevus of Ota. Periodic ophthalmologic exams are clearly warranted in patients with this disease.

DIFFERENTIAL DIAGNOSIS: Mongolian Spot. Although it presents at birth and is commonly located in the lumbosacral region, Mongolian Spots usually do not persist into adulthood.

TREATMENT OPTIONS: The Q-switched ruby laser is an effective treatment for unresolved lesions.

PALMOPLANTAR HYPERPIGMENTATION

Polymorphous, hyperpigmented macules on the plantar surfaces may cause confusion with secondary syphilis. However, the benign pigmentation pictured lacks the surface scale often associated with syphilis.

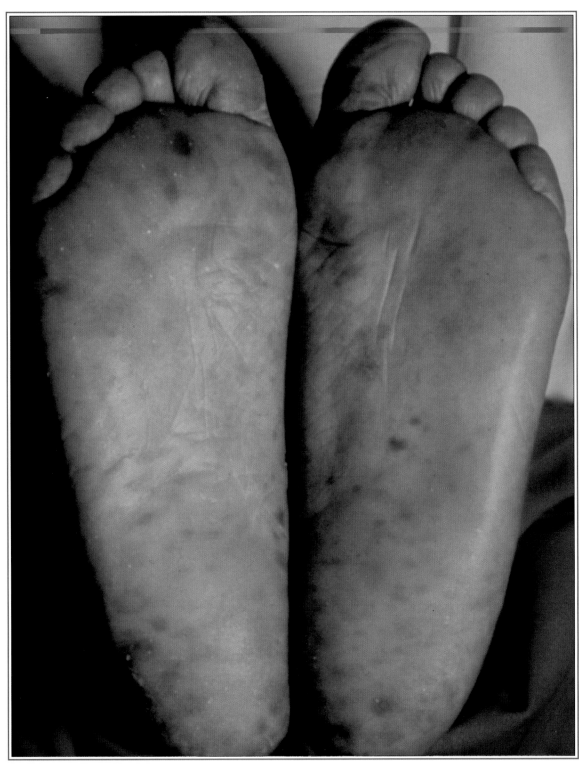

DEFINITION: Palmoplantar Hyperpigmentation is a common variant found in black people.

ETIOLOGY: The hyperpigmentation is the result of localized hypermelanosis. The more heavily pigmented an individual, the more likely one finds this condition.

CLINICAL PERSPECTIVE: These polymorphous brown macules may have sharp or indistinct borders. Multiple lesions without surface changes are normal.

DIFFERENTIAL DIAGNOSIS: The pigmented Palmoplantar lesions of secondary syphilis may mimic the normal variant. However, the lesions of syphilis tend to be monomorphous and have a predilection for the palms and arches of the feet.

TREATMENT: Therapeutic intervention is not necessary. The condition is benign.

PITYRIASIS ALBA

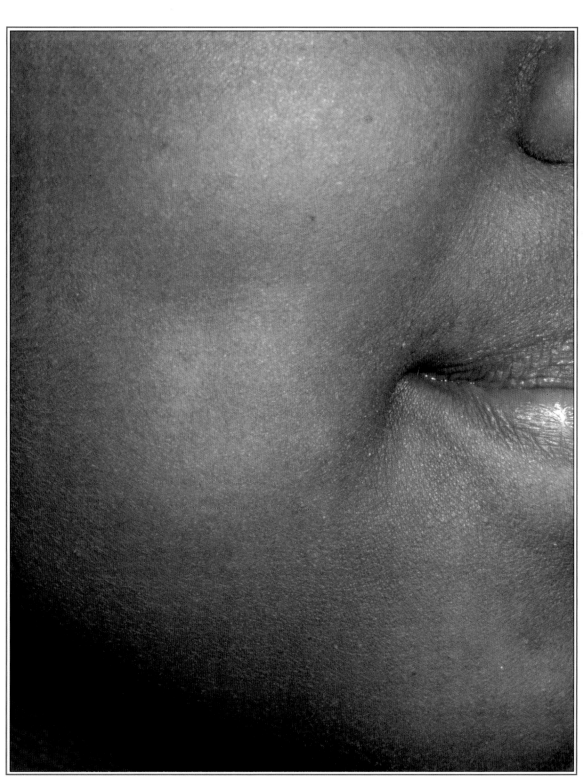

Hypopigmented patches on the cheek of a 10-year-old female are characteristic of pityriasis alba. The patient's mother stated that reddish, scaling lesions had preceded the current dermatosis.

DEFINITION: Pityriasis Alba consists of scaling, erythematous papules which evolve into 5-30 mm hypopigmented patches.

ETIOLOGY: Pityriasis Alba is believed to be a variant of atopic dermatitis. The hypopigmented patches result from a decrease in the number of active melanocytes. Some researchers, however, believe the hypopigmentation may be due to a reduced capacity of the epidermal cells to acquire melanin during an inflammatory process. Black children aged three to sixteen are most likely to develop this condition, although adult cases have been reported.

CLINICAL PERSPECTIVE: The disease is usually confined to the face, although approximately 20% of affected children will have neck, arm and shoulder involvement. The initial papules are often barely noticeable. It is the residual hypopigmentation which leads patients or their families to seek medical consultation.

DIFFERENTIAL DIAGNOSIS: Vitiligo is depigmented and located periorifically. Pityriasis Alba is hypopigmented and usually found on the malar region.

TREATMENT OPTIONS: The erythematous scaling phase of Pityriasis Alba may be treated with non-fluorinated topical corticosteroids. Emollient cream or mild tar paste may also be tried. For post-inflammatory hypopigmentation, 0.1% 8-methoxypsoralen with short exposures to UVA (0.25-0.50J) once or twice weekly may be attempted. Oral psoralens plus UVA exposure (PUVA) has been proven effective in treating widespread disease in adults.

PITYRIASIS ROSEA

TOP

Slightly scaling, oval, hyperpigmented papules on the trunk suggest a diagnosis of pityriasis rosea. The larger, scaling 'herald patch' on the shoulder preceded the generalized eruption by three weeks. This precursor lesion is virtually pathognomonic for pityriasis rosea.

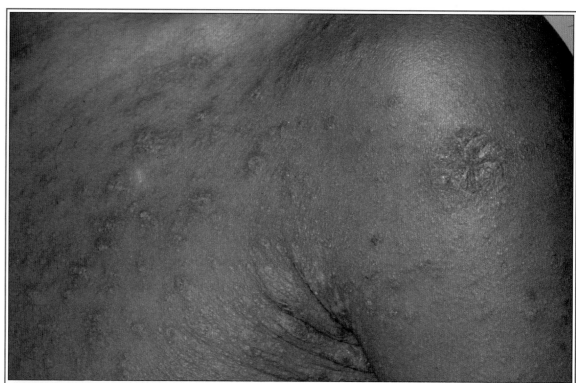

LOWER

A 35-year-old male with reddish brown oval papules on the posterior thorax and dorsal arms. The lesions of pityriasis rosea follow the skin cleavage lines in a 'Christmas tree' distribution.

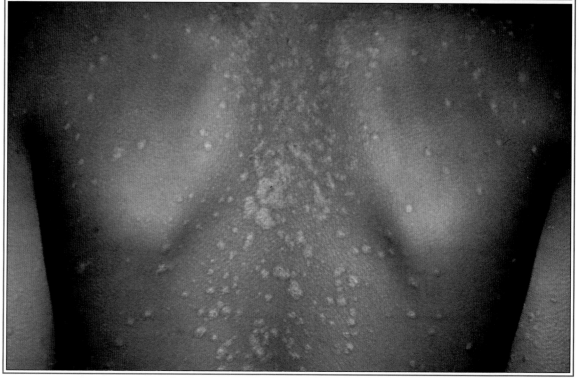

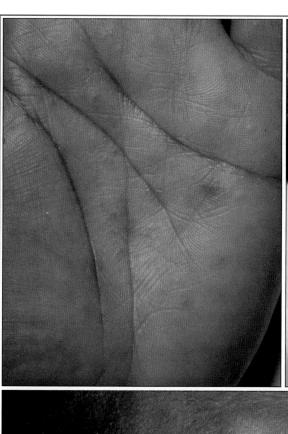

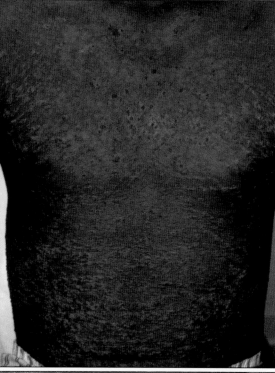

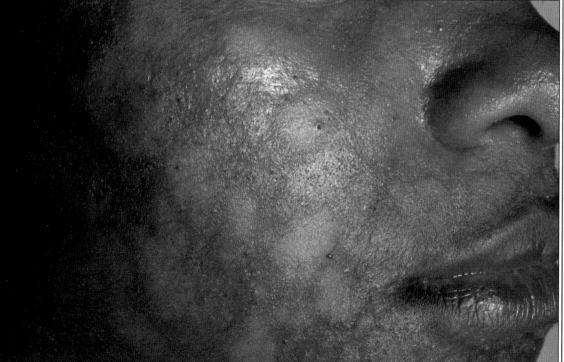

TOP

This 45-year-old female demonstrates the papulovesicular form of pityriasis rosea more frequently encountered among black people. Many 2-3 mm reddish-brown papulovisicles are found on the dorsal hand and proximal fingers of this patient.

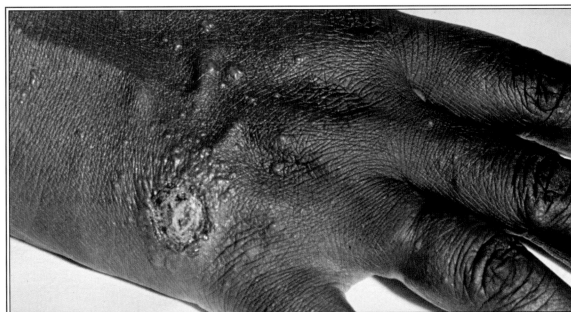

LOWER RIGHT

Close-up view of a 17-year-old male with large, scaling patches of pityriasis rosea on the chest. This case reveals the distinctive scaling form of pityriasis rosea found in black patients.

LOWER LEFT

A scaling form of pityriasis rosea is seen in black people. This 17-year-old male has widespread oval coalescing scaling patches on the anterior thorax and upper arms.

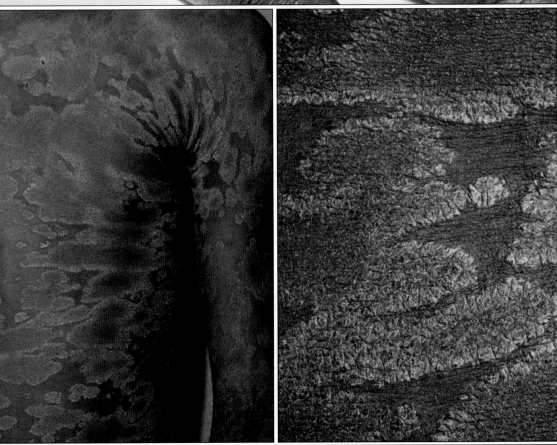

DEFINITION: Pityriasis Rosea consists of oval papules with a marginal scale that follow the skin cleavage lines. A larger scaling patch (herald patch), may precede the generalized eruption.

ETIOLOGY: The etiology is unknown, although a viral cause has been proposed. A seasonal occurrence (spring - autumn), limited 6-8 week course, and the presence of a primary lesion evolving into a secondary eruption are consistent with a viral disease.

CLINICAL PERSPECTIVE: Pityriasis Rosea takes on peculiar variations in black skin. Instead of the classic salmon colored papules ascribed to Caucasian skin, a reddish brown-gray color is normally visable. A papulovesicular or papular form with prominent scale may also be encountered. The lesions are usually distributed on the trunk in a 'christmas tree' pattern. However, an inverse distribution involving the face, lower abdomen and extremities is not uncommon in black people. Black patients have an increased recurrence rate of approximately 6%, which is nearly double the rate found in Caucasians.

DIFFERENTIAL DIAGNOSIS: Secondary syphilis may closely mimic Pityriasis Rosea. Serum RPR levels should be obtained if the diagnosis is in doubt and a careful history should aid in the diagnosis of drug eruptions. Guttate psoriasis often follows a streptococcal infection and tends to have a thicker white scale.

TREATMENT OPTIONS: Treatment is usually unnecessary due to the self-limited nature of the disease. In pruritic or widespread cases, topical or intramuscular corticosteroids may alleviate the pruritis and reduce the likelihood of post-inflammatory hyperpigmentation. Ultraviolet B light (UVB) treatment, particularly during the first week of therapy, can be helpful in diffuse or symptomatic cases.

POMADE ACNE

Pomade acne consists of multiple comedones and reddish papules on the forehead. The adult female shown opposite has applied oils to her scalp for years. Discontinuation of the oils led to complete resolution.

DEFINITION: Comedones at the site of prolonged hair oil application lead to the condition called Pomade Acne.

ETIOLOGY: Due the inherently curved hairs in black people, the natural scalp oils often fail to reach terminal hair shafts. As a result, hair becomes dry and brittle which necessitates the use of lubricating pomades comprised of comedogenic paraffins and petrolatum. Pomade Acne has a predilection for adults, although children may adopt the hair care techniques of their elders and subsequently develop this condition.

CLINICAL PERSPECTIVE: The comedones ('white heads', 'black heads') usually involve the forehead and temples. Inflammatory papules may occur to a lesser degree. The scalp often appears greasy due to the pomades.

DIFFERENTIAL DIAGNOSIS: The primary lesion of acne vulgaris is also a comedone. Papules, pustules or cysts may also be found. Acne vulgaris is generally not limited to the forehead. A history of pomade application will aid in the diagnosis.

TREATMENT OPTIONS: Treatment consists of pomade avoidance and the reduction of greasy comedogenic oils.

POST-INFLAMMATORY HYPER/HYPOPIGMENTATION

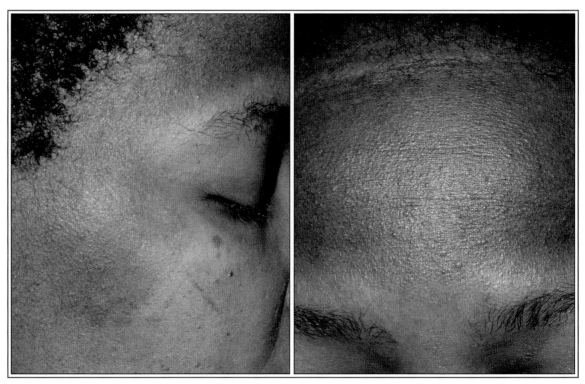

Post-inflammatory hyperpigmentation in a 39-year-old female secondary to contact dermatitis from perfume. This condition lacks surface changes, i.e., scale.

DEFINITION: Black skin may respond to inflammatory disease or trauma by either an increase or decrease in pigmentation.

ETIOLOGY: Diseases characteristically associated with hyperpigmentation include: acne vulgaris, atopic dermatitis, contact dermatitis, fixed drug eruption, pityriasis rosea, lichen planus, secondary syphilis, sarcoidosis and mycosis fungoides. Diseases which may be associated with hypopigmentation include: atopic dermatitis, contact dermatitis, seborrheic dermatitis, pityriasis alba, discoid lupus erythematosus, sarcoidosis, scleroderma, lichen striatus, secondary syphilis and mycosis fungoides. Almost any inflammatory disease presented in black people may resolve and still lead to hyperpigmentation or hypopigmentation. For example, acne vulgaris, even if properly treated often leaves pigmentation. This appearance may be distressing to patients who may think their

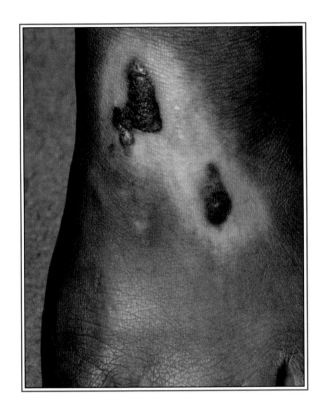

Long term ultra-potent topical corticosteroids applied to the ankle caused post-inflammatory hypopigmentation in this patient. Normal pigmentation eventually returned following discontinuation of the offending agent.

treatment regimen is failing and patient reassurance is required. Preventing new lesions should be the physician's goal. Physical modalities such as cryosurgery, laser surgery and dermabrasion may also lead to hypopigmentation or hyperpigmentation. Topical, intralesional and intramuscular corticosteroids (particularly fluorinated steroids) may cause undesirable hypopigmentation in black people.

CLINICAL PERSPECTIVE: Post-inflammatory hyper/hypopigmentation is more noticeable in black people. Patience should be emphasized with these individuals since many pigmentary alterations normalize with time.

DIFFERENTIAL DIAGNOSIS: A thorough search for the primary cutaneous lesion, if present, will establish the diagnosis. The patient will often provide the details of the original condition leading to pigmentary alterations.

TREATMENT OPTIONS: Post-inflammatory Hypopigmentation will often repigment and fade over time. Dilute (0.1%) 8-methoxypsoralen and low doses of ultraviolet A (PUVA) may be used to hasten the repigmentation. Topical tretinoin 0.1% cream, azelaic acid and hydroquinone cream can aid in the treatment of the hyperpigmentation.

PSEUDOFOLLICULITIS BARBAE

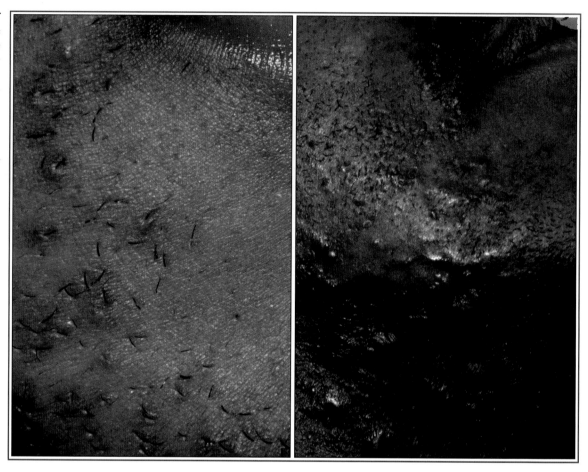

DEFINITION: Pseudofolliculitis Barbae occurs when ingrown hairs create a foreign body reaction. This prevalent condition primarily affects black males.

ETIOLOGY: Shaving curved hairs leads to transfollicular and extrafollicular penetration. During transfollicular penetration, the inherently curved hair shaft pierces the follicle creating a dermal foreign body reaction. Pulling the hair taut prior to shaving permits the shaft to retract beneath the skin surface, further exacerbating this condition. Extrafollicular penetration arises when the hair shaft moves up through the epidermis only to curve downward and re-enter the integument.

CLINICAL PERSPECTIVE: The primary lesion consists of a firm papule often containing a hair remnant. Secondary lesions in the form of pustules are common. Scarring, keloids, hyperpigmentation and infection with Staphylococcal aureus represent potential secondary changes. While the beard region is the most common site, other shaved areas, including the groin and scalp, may be involved.

DIFFERENTIAL DIAGNOSIS: Bacterial folliculitis (sycosis barbae) consists of small pustules often affecting the upper lip. Dermatophyte folliculitis (tinea barbae) is often located on the chin or submaxillary region and rarely involves the upper lip. Bacterial and fungal cultures will aid in the diagnosis.

TREATMENT OPTIONS: A number of treatments can be employed. Beard growth for one month permits the ingrown hairs to become extruded. A Pseudofolliculitis Barbae razor and electric clippers can trim hair lengths to 1 mm or greater. This ideal hair length makes hair entrapment less likely. Chemical depilatories containing barium sulfide permit a smooth shave but leave a sulfur odor. Alternatively, calcium thioglycolate depilatories have a more tolerable mercaptan odor but provide a less smooth shave. Shelly [195] recommends that the patient should not (1) pull the skin taut for a closer shave, (2) shave against the grain or (3) shave back and forth over the same area. Glycolic acid peels, beginning at lower strength and repeated monthly, provide improvement. Tretinoin cream and glycolic acid lotion may be helpful. Corticosteroid lotion applied after shaving reduces inflammation. An aggressive surgical approach for refractory cases of Pseudofolliculitis Barbae has been suggested by Bouman [185]. The procedure involves making an incision, everting the skin, cutting the hair roots and finally extraction. Antibiotics may be necessary to treat secondary infection and for the anti-inflammatory effect.

Psoriasis Vulgaris

Multiple gray-violaceous well demarcated plaques on the forehead, temple, and cheek of an 18-year-old male with psoriasis. The lesions resolved after administration of topical corticosteroids. However, post-inflammatory hyperpigmentation lasted many months. Facial involvement is uncommon.

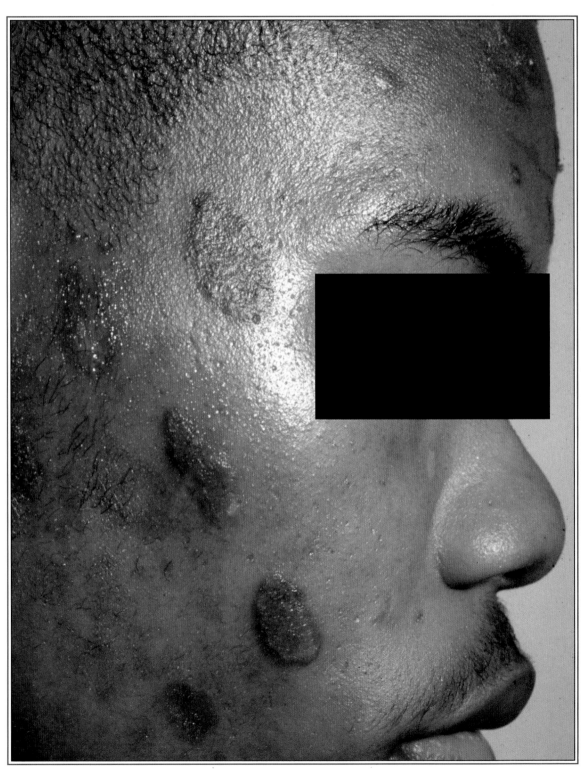

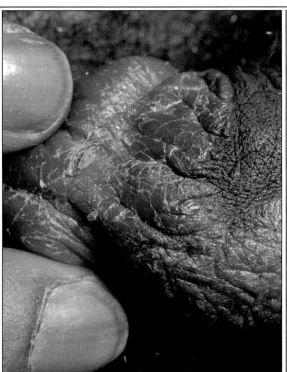

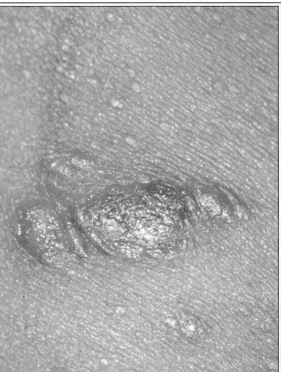

TOP LEFT

A 28-year-old male with scaling, gray-violaceous plaques in another common location, the penis.

TOP RIGHT

A 28-year-old female with a violaceous, slightly scaling 30 mm psoriatic plaque of the abdomen. Multiple, discrete, firm slightly scaling 2-5 mm violaceous papules are also scattered throughout the abdomen. This papular form of psoriasis may also be found in black patients.

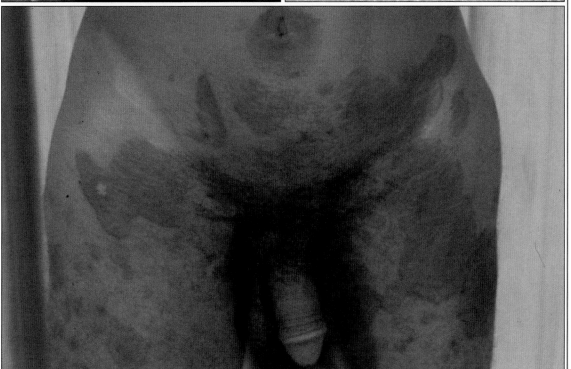

LOWER

Psoriasis has a predilection for certain anatomical sites including the extensor surfaces of the arms and legs and the umbilicus as found on this 23-year-old male. Note the gray-violaceous color of the slightly scaling plaques which lack the brick red color typical of psoriasis in Caucasians.

TOP
This 45-year-old male has many of the nail changes associated with psoriasis. The affected nails are dystrophic and exhibit small pits.

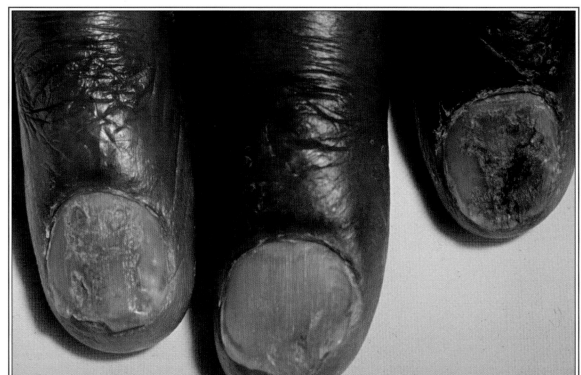

LOWER
Grayish-tan, hyperkeratotic, well demarcated plaques in a periumbilical distribution represent psoriasis in this 44-year-old black female. The erythematous plaques usually found in Caucasians are often absent in black people.

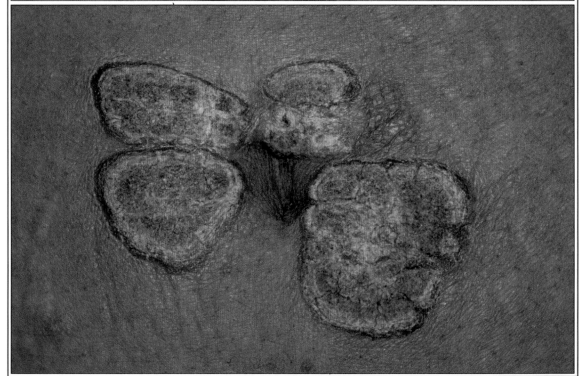

DEFINITION: An inflammatory disease with increased production of epidermal cells resulting in an increase in the stratum corneum.

ETIOLOGY: The cause of Psoriasis Vulgaris is unknown. Approximately 1% of the U.S. population and about 2% of European Caucasians are affected. The disease is less common in black people of West African and African American descent.

CLINICAL PERSPECTIVE: The lesions of Psoriasis Vulgaris are sharply demarcated, erythematous papules and plaques covered by a silvery white scale. Sites of predilection include the scalp, extensor elbows and knees, umbilicus and the lumbosacral region. Nail involvement in the form of pits, subungual debris and the 'oil-mark' sign is common in Caucasians. Nail changes are less often found in black people. Psoriasis may appear differently in black people. The typical erythematous, micaceous scaling plaques can assume a violaceous or deep blue color. Post-inflammatory hyperpigmentation often causes concern among black patients with Psoriasis.

DIFFERENTIAL DIAGNOSIS: Other papulosquamous diseases including lichen planus, pityriasis rosea, tinea versicolor, pityriasis lichenoides chronica, tinea corporis, drug eruptions, and secondary syphilis may resemble Psoriasis.

TREATMENT OPTIONS: Topical emollients, tars, corticosteroids, and calcipotriol are useful treatments for Psoriasis Vulgaris. Light therapy (UVB, PUVA) and systemic medications such as methotrexate and etretinate may be necessary.

SARCOIDOSIS

TOP LEFT

Ulcerative sarcoidosis is almost exclusive to the black population. Pictured here are multiple, punched out, 8-15 mm, peripherally hyperpigmented ulcers on the leg of a 45-year-old female.

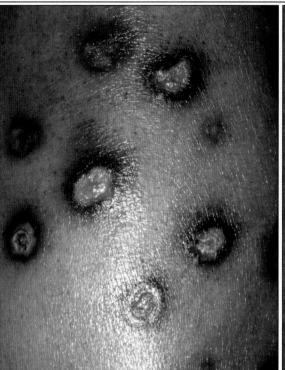

TOP RIGHT

A biopsy of this annular, reddish-brown plaque with central hypopigmentation revealed cutaneous sarcoidosis. Hypopigmented patches and annular configurations are frequently encountered in black patients with this disease.

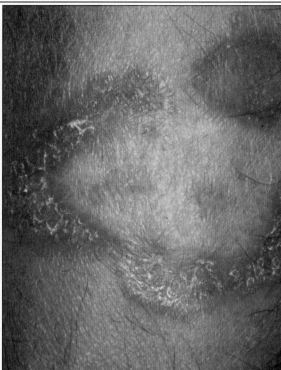

LOWER

Numerous, reddish-brown, 2-3 mm waxy papules of cutaneous sarcoidosis involving the periocular region of a 27-year-old nurse. These firm, waxy papules represent the most common specific type of cutaneous sarcoidosis among black patients.

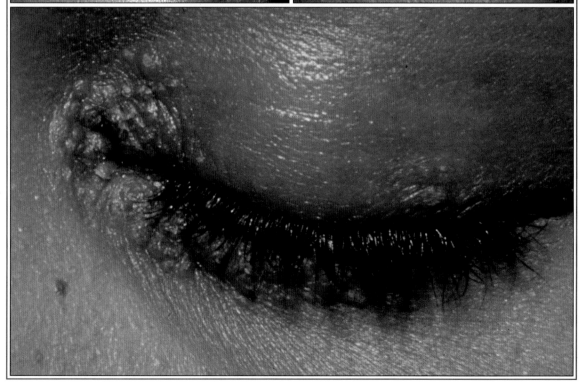

DEFINITION: Sarcoidosis is a multisystem granulomatous disease with cutaneous involvement in 10% to 30% of patients. Sarcoidosis is ten times more common in black people and may carry a worse prognosis.

ETIOLOGY: The etiology of Sarcoidosis is unknown.

CLINICAL PERSPECTIVE: One will find two types of lesions which are specific and non-specific. The specific lesions demonstrate non-caseating granulomas on histological examination. Reddish-brown or slightly hypopigmented, waxy papules are the most common specific lesions found on black skin. Sites of predilection include the perinasal, periorbital and melolabial areas. Hypopigmented macules and psoriasiform lesions are more frequently encountered in this ethnic group. Lupus pernio lesions (consisting of violaceous papules and plaques usually located on the nose, malar region, or ears) are less commonly found in black patients. Annular, icthyosiform and ulcerative Sarcoidosis are almost exclusive to the black population. Subcutaneous Sarcoidosis (Darier-Roussy sarcoid), consisting of nodules located on the trunk and extremities, has also been documented.

The most common non-specific Sarcoidal form is erythema nodosum. About 2% of all black people develop this manifestation. These tender, reddish nodules are often found on the anterior lower legs and are believed to represent a type of hypersensitivity reaction.

DIFFERENTIAL DIAGNOSIS: Papular mucinosis, lichen amyloidosis, generalized granuloma annulare, lupus vulgaris and secondary syphilis may resemble cutaneous sarcoidosis. A biopsy can confirm the diagnosis.

TREATMENT OPTIONS: Topical, intralesional and oral corticosteroids, as well as antimalarials, may be necessary to control the disease.

SEBORRHEIC DERMATITIS

TOP LEFT

Seborrheic dermatitis: A 27-year-old female with hypopigmented, scaling patches of the forehead and eyebrows. When the anterior hair line shows this distinctive hypopigmentation, a diagnosis of seborrheic dermatitis can be made from across the examination room.

TOP RIGHT

Impetigo, a bacterial infection, reveals honey colored crusts.

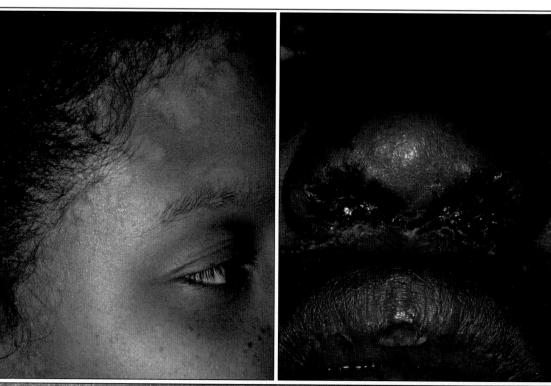

LOWER

The eyebrows are commonly affected in seborrheic dermatitis. Reddish scaling papules with hypopigmentation are evident. A short course of topical corticosteroids and antifungals are often curative.

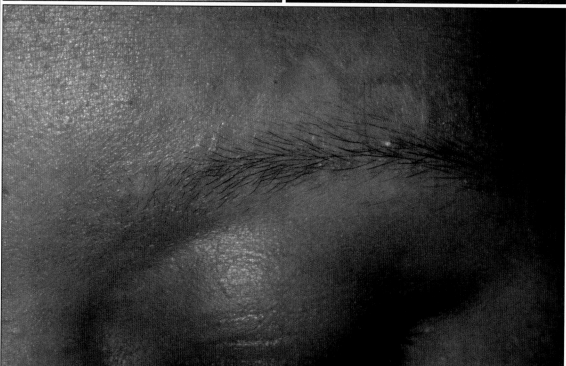

DEFINITION: This common, chronic inflammatory disease involves the scalp, eyebrows, melolabial folds, ears, and presternal regions.

ETIOLOGY: The cause is unknown. Large numbers of the yeast Pityrosporum ovale are found on the scalp. The question of whether this organism causes seborrheic dermatitis is a matter of debate. The incidence of Seborrheic Dermatitis is increased in HIV infected individuals.

CLINICAL PERSPECTIVE: In infants, a greasy, yellow scale is seen most often on the scalp ('cradle cap') or intertriginous folds. Adults demonstrate a white or yellowish scale with erythema located on the scalp, eyebrows, melolabial folds, ears and sternal regions.

Post-inflammatory hypopigmentation is often a problem in darker pigmented patients. This hypopigmentation may be further exacerbated by topical corticosteroids used to treat the Seborrheic Dermatitis. The hypopigmentation is commonly found on the anterior hairline, eyebrows and melolabial folds in black adults. Once the dermatitis is treated, the post-inflammatory hypopigmentation will gradually return to normal.

DIFFERENTIAL DIAGNOSIS: Atopic dermatitis (positive family history, hayfever, asthma, eczema, pruritic, flexural distribution); psoriasis (less common on face, thick white scale); contact dermatitis (erythematous or vesicular, history); impetigo (honey colored crusts).

TREATMENT OPTIONS: Anti-seborrheic shampoos (selenium sulfide, zinc pyrithion, ketoconazole), Salicylic acid (removes scale), and low-to-mid potency corticosteroids for a limited duration are beneficial. Antifungal creams may also be effective.

SICKLE CELL LEG ULCERS

LEFT

Tender sickle cell ulcers are commonly found near the maleolus. Wound dressings which promoted a moist environment, antibiotics and pentoxifylline led to healing in this recalcitrant ulcer.

RIGHT

A well demarcated 'punched out' ulcer on the lower legs of a black patient should alert the physician to the possibility of sickle cell disease.

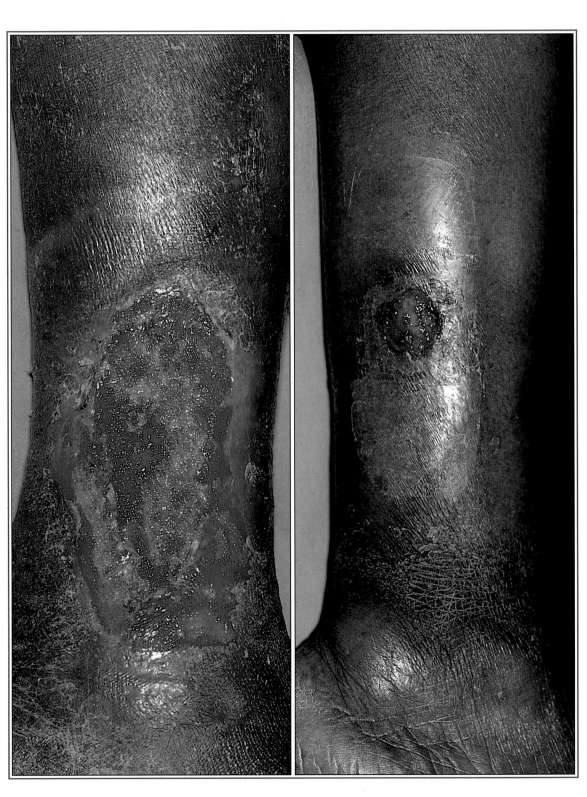

DEFINITION: Approximately 10% of African Americans are heterozygous for the sickle cell gene. Leg ulcers represent the most frequent cutaneous finding in black people with sickle cell disease and 25-75% of homozygous sickle cell patients develop lower leg ulcers. Young adults are mostly affected, with rare occurrences under the age of fifteen.

ETIOLOGY: Vaso-occlusion, infection and trauma represent mechanisms by which Sickle Cell Ulcers may develop. Venous insufficiency does not appear to be a factor in the pathogenesis. Microflora such as Staphylococcus aureus, Pseudomonas, Group A Streptococcus and Corynebacterium diptheriae have all been isolated from the ulcer base and these organisms contribute to poor wound healing, inflammation and local lymphadenopathy.

CLINICAL PERSPECTIVE: The Sickle Cell Ulcers are usually located near the malleoli. Single and multiple types exist with a unilateral or bilateral distribution. Pain is a common feature.

DIFFERENTIAL DIAGNOSIS: Table 2 provides an analysis of lower extremity ulcers.

TREATMENT OPTIONS: Treatments for Sickle Cell Leg Ulcers include topical antibiotics, flagyl and bed rest. Recombinant human erythropoietin has been shown to increase ulcer healing time and topical synthetic extracellular matrix accelerates the healing process. Skin and muscle grafting may eventually be necessary.

SYPHILIS

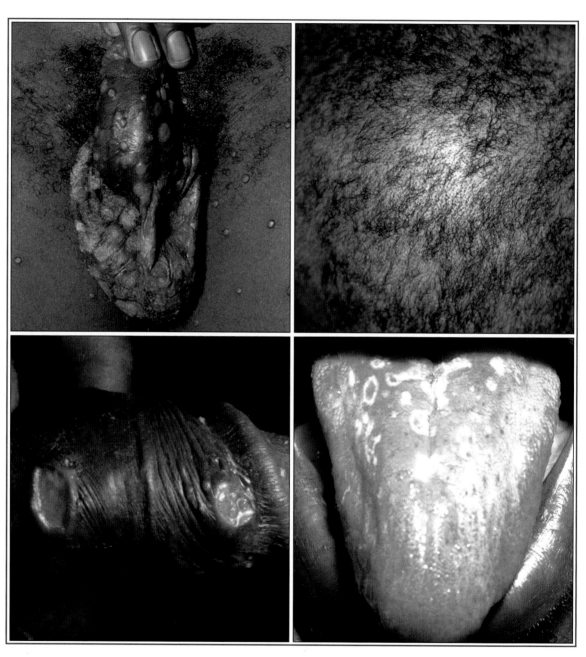

DEFINITION: Syphilis is a sexually transmitted disease known as the 'great imitator' due to its polymorphous clinical presentations. Many would argue, however, that HIV has become the new 'great imitator'.

ETIOLOGY: The spirochete *Treponema Pallidum* is the causative organism.

CLINICAL PERSPECTIVE: Several distinct clinical variations of syphilitic lesions have been noted in black people. While a macular syphilid is common in Caucasians, follicular, papular and pustular forms are more frequent in the black community. A perioral annular form of secondary Syphilis is almost exclusive to black people. These distinctive lesions are known as 'nickles and dimes' since they present as coin-like hyperpigmented patches. Hyperkeratotic palmoplantar lesions, the so-called lues cornee, must be differentiated from normal palmoplantar hyperpigmentation. A helpful clue to the correct diagnosis is that the lues cornee lesions tend to be monomorphous and involve the mid-plantar surface.

A patchy alopecia is more common in black patients with secondary syphilis. This non-scarring alopecia has been described as 'moth eaten'. Moist, flat papules in the intertriginous regions known as condyloma lata are commonly seen in black females with syphilis. Gummas, a form of tertiary Syphilis, are six times more frequent in black people than Caucasians. These lesions are granulomatous and often ulcerate.

DIFFERENTIAL DIAGNOSIS: Other papulosquamous diseases, including pityriasis rosea, psoriasis, atopic dermatitis, drug eruption, tinea versicolor, tinea corporis, pityriasis lichenoides chronica, and mycosis fungoides may simulate secondary Syphilis. When the diagnosis is in doubt, a serum RPR is warranted.

TREATMENT OPTIONS: Primary, secondary, or early Syphilis is successfully treated with intramuscular penicillin G 2.4 million U in a single dose. The same dose repeated weekly for three consecutive weeks is needed to treat Syphilis of indeterminate length or more than one year's duration.

TOP LEFT

Numerous, reddish, moist papules coalescing to plaques in the perianal region of a 20-year-old female with condyloma lata.

TOP RIGHT

Primary syphilis often presents with a solitary, indurated, painless erosion as seen on the distal penile shaft of this 18-year-old male. T.pallidum may be demonstrated on dark field microscopic examination from lesional scrapings.

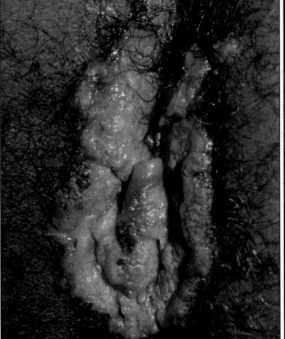
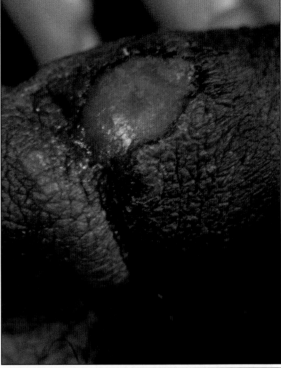

LOWER LEFT

A 48-year-old construction worker with numerous, tan, discrete and confluent papules of the posterior thorax and arms. This papular form of secondary syphilis is more common in black people.

LOWER RIGHT

Flesh colored 2-7 mm papules on the dorsal aspects of the feet in this 20-year-old male attest to the distinctive papular nature of secondary syphilis in black people.

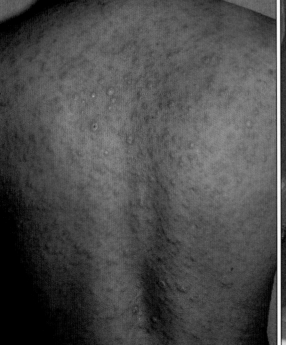
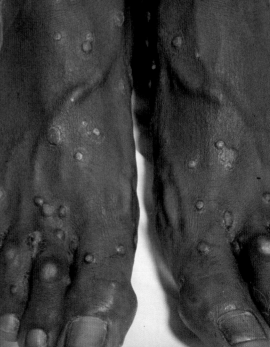

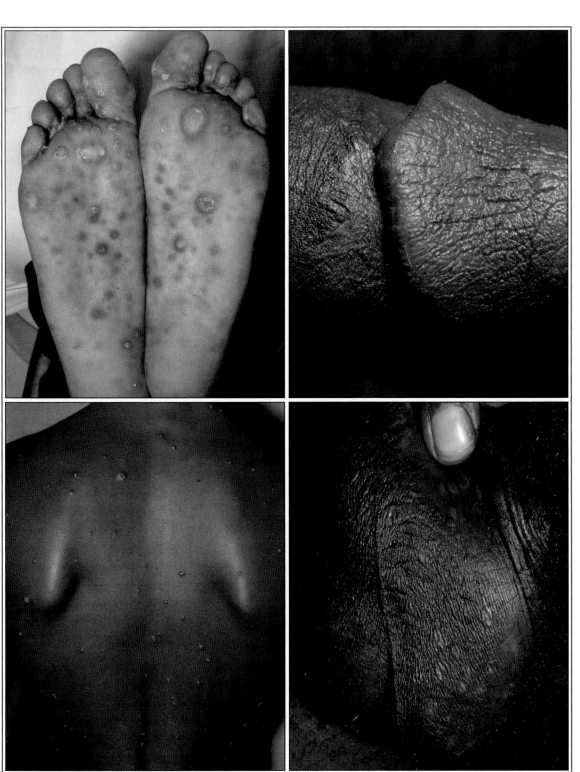

TINEA CAPITIS

TOP LEFT

Close up views illustrating the white scale typical of tinea capitis in black patients. The similarity of the scale to seborrheic dermatitis often requires a fungal culture or KOH preparation to distinguish the two conditions.

TOP ABOVE RIGHT

The grandmother of this 7-year-old male was concerned that his hair would never return. Physical examination shows diffuse scale with loss of scalp hair. The correct diagnosis is tinea capitis.

TOP BELOW RIGHT

The same patient (as above right) after receiving an eight week course of an oral antifungal. Both grandmother and patient were relieved when hair growth resumed, and inflammation subsided.

LOWER LEFT

This large, boggy, purulent plaque on the occipital scalp of a 12-year-old male is an example of a kerion. Kerions represent an inflammatory response to tinea infection.

LOWER RIGHT

A 12-year-old male presented with a well circumscribed, non-scaling patch of hair loss of the anterior scalp. This case of alopecia areata, lacks the surface scale seen in tinea capitis. Furthermore, small proximally tapered 'exclamation point hairs' may be found in the patches of alopecia areata.

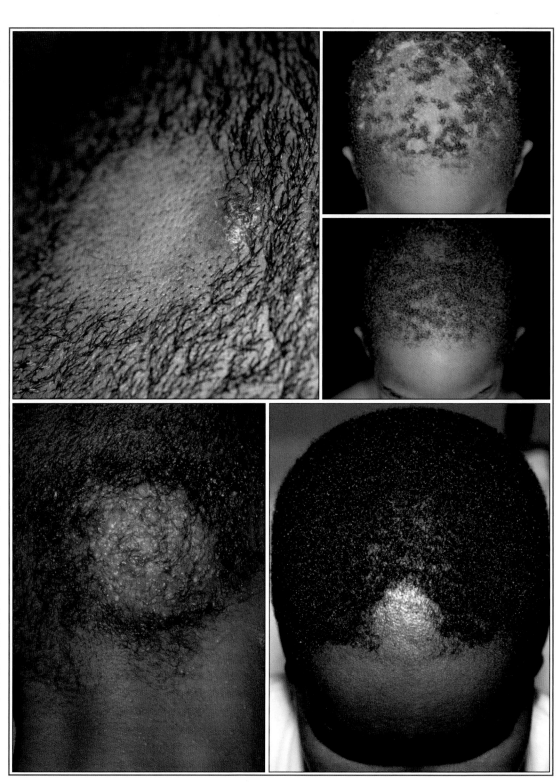

DEFINITION: Dermatophyte infection of the hair shaft causes Tinea Capitis. Tinea Capitis caused by different dermatophyte species varies according to geographical distribution. See Table 3.

ETIOLOGY: *Trichophyton tonsurans* has replaced *Microsporum audouinii* as the main fungal organism responsible for Tinea Capitis in the United States and represents over 90% of all cases. Before the 1950s , *Microsporum audouinii* was largely responsible for Tinea Capitis in the United States and Europe. *T. tonsurans* is highly infectious and is spread via person to person contact. Transfer of infection from brushes, combs, theater seats and linen has been reported. Most of these cases involve black children. Investigators have speculated that tight braiding may make it easier for the fungus to invade the exposed stratum corneum. The use of pomades in black children may allow the spore to remain tightly attached to the hair until a penetrating fungal hypha is formed.

CLINICAL PERSPECTIVE: Tinea Capitis caused by *T. tonsurans* may present as a patch of broken hairs at the skin surface, the so-called 'black dot' form. Some scaling or erythema may be present. Often, only a slight grayish-white scale with minimal hair loss is demonstrated. This appearance may cause confusion with seborrheic dermatitis.

DIFFERENTIAL DIAGNOSIS: Seborrheic dermatitis may resemble Tinea Capitis caused by *T. tonsurans*. When in doubt, a fungal culture or KOH preparation will aid in the diagnosis. Psoriasis, alopecia areata, impetigo, pediculosis capitis, trichotillomania, and secondary syphilis may be included in the differential diagnosis.

TREATMENT OPTIONS: Oral antifungals in conjunction with topical antifungal shampoos will cure the disease.

TINEA VERSICOLOR

TOP LEFT

Grayish-brown scaling patches of tinea versicolor in a 25-year-old male. Note the follicular, discrete and confluent scaling papules of the posterior neck. This follicular pattern is more common in black patients with this disorder.

TOP RIGHT

The same patient, as top left, demonstrates the distinctive gray-brown follicular scaling papules of tinea versicolor on the anterior neck and chest. In contrast, Caucasians with tinea versicolor exhibit fawn colored patches.

LOWER LEFT

This 17-year-old female was distressed due to cosmetically objectionable hypopigmented macules and patches occurring on the eyebrows and cheeks. Hypopigmented tinea versicolor is common in black people. The facial distribution shows that lesions may be found on areas other than the characteristic truncal locations.

LOWER RIGHT

A 34-year-old female with multiple, discrete, and coalescing hypopigmented 3-20 mm patches along the chin and mandibular region. A vigorous scratch of the examining nail will produce the furfuraceous scale characteristic of tinea versicolor. Post-inflammatory hypopigmentation may persist in black people with tinea versicolor and cause cosmetic concern.

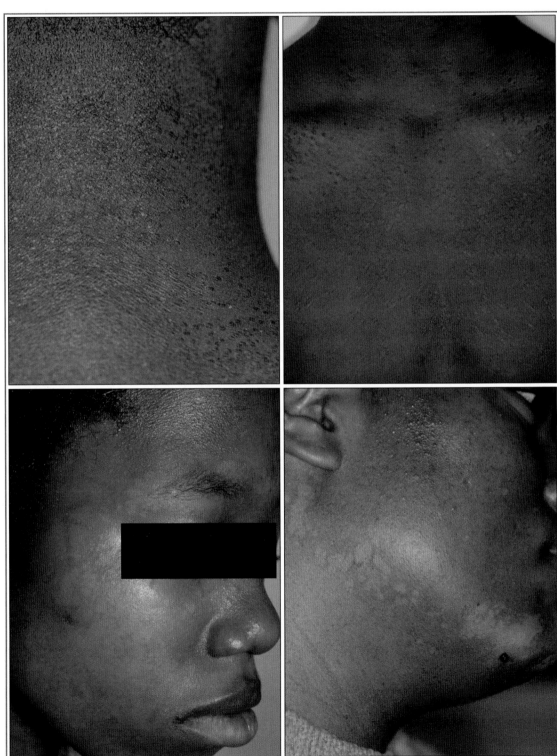

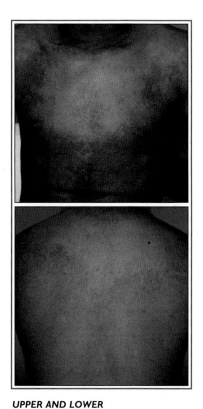

UPPER AND LOWER

Confluent and reticulate papillomatosis of the chest and back in a 24-year-old male may mimic tinea versicolor. These flat hyperpigmented papules become partially confluent at their periphery forming a reticulate pattern. This condition is considered to be due to a defect in keratinization although the yeast, Pityrosporum orbiculare has been demonstrated in some cases.

DEFINITION: Tinea Versicolor is a common papulosquamous disease which favors the trunk and shoulders.

ETIOLOGY: The causative agent is the yeast-like organism, Pityrosporum orbiculare. Tinea Versicolor flourishes in tropical climates and is found more frequently among black people residing in these areas.

CLINICAL PERSPECTIVE: Fawn colored patches with a furfuraceous (dust-like) scale are described in Caucasians but Tinea Versicolor appears as gray-brown hyperpigmented, scaly patches in black patients. The sternal region, sides of chest, abdomen, back and neck are often involved. Occasionally, follicular or hypopigmented lesions are seen.

DIFFERENTIAL DIAGNOSIS: Seborrheic dermatitis (yellow greasy scales), pityriasis rosea (papules with collarette scale, follow skin lines), and syphilis (palms and soles frequently involved with positive RPR) must be differentiated from Tinea Versicolor. A yellow or brown colored fluorescence under Wood's light is a helpful diagnostic clue in this disease.

TREATMENT OPTIONS: Oral and topical antifungals or selenium sulfide 2.5% suspension are highly curative.

TRACTION ALOPECIA

TOP

Tight braids have led to temporal hair loss in this young adult female.

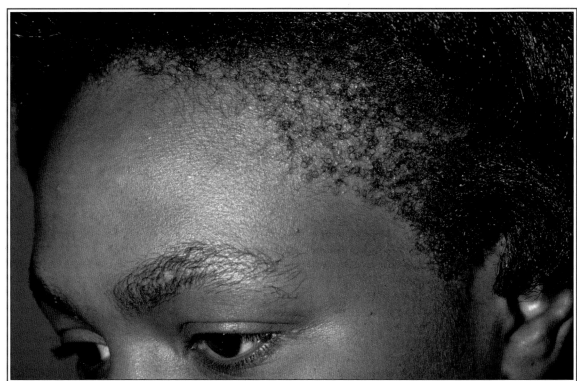

LOWER

Exaggerated hair loss is evident in this young girl who styled her hair in tight 'corn rows'. Note the shortened hairs distal to the patch of hair loss, a clue to the correct diagnosis of traction alopecia.

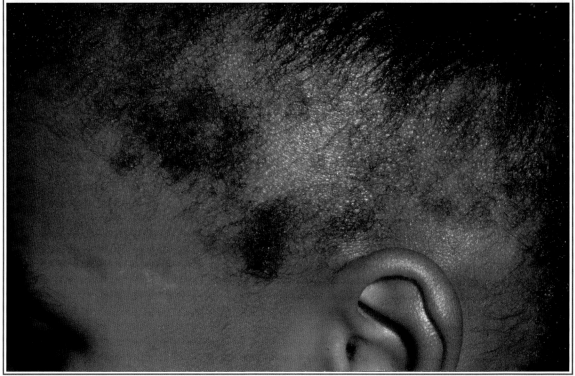

DEFINITION: Gradual hair loss due to prolonged tension on the scalp gives rise to Traction Alopecia.

ETIOLOGY: Hot combs, tight hair braids, bands, and rollers have been implicated in the pathogenesis. Contracting facial muscles may exacerbate the temporoparietal alopecia.

CLINICAL PERSPECTIVE: Erythema and follicular pustules represent early lesions, whereas atrophy and cicatricial alopecia are late sequelae. The distribution varies but usually involves the vertex and temporoparietal areas. Shortened hairs distal to the affected area provide a useful diagnostic clue.

DIFFERENTIAL DIAGNOSIS: Alopecia areata and trichotillomania may closely resemble Traction Alopecia. Alopecia areata consists of round or diffuse areas of hair loss with 'exclamation point hairs'. Trichotillomania involves hairs of varying lengths.

TREATMENT OPTIONS: Treatment is based on prevention. However, due to long standing hair care practices, this advice may be dismissed by the patient. Oral and topical antibiotics are useful for the erythema and pustules. Hair transplantation may be necessary for alopecia of long duration.

VITILIGO

TOP LEFT

Note the white atrophic patches occurring on the temporal scalp and inner ear of a 39-year-old male with discoid lupus erythematosus. The inner ear is a frequent location of discoid lupus erythematosus in black people. Another important diagnostic feature of discoid lupus erythematosus in black persons is the presence of perilesional hyperpigmentation.

TOP RIGHT

The depigmented patches of vitiligo are often found on the hands.

LOWER LEFT

Discoid lupus erythematosus of the scalp may lead to a scarring alopecia. This 8 cm hypopigmented patch on the scalp of a 40-year-old female can mimic vitiligo. However, vitiligo lacks the atrophy, follicular plugging and adherent scale of discoid lupus erythematosus.

LOWER RIGHT

This 22-year-old secretary has well demarcated depigmented patches on the dorsal aspects of her fingers consistent with a diagnosis of vitiligo. The 'white spots' were cosmetically objectionable to this young woman.

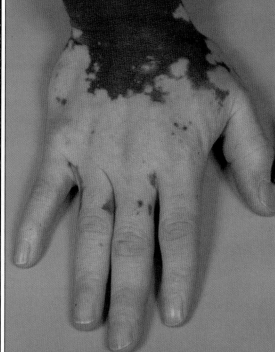

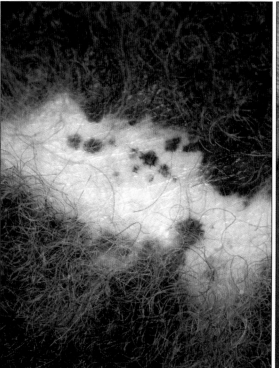

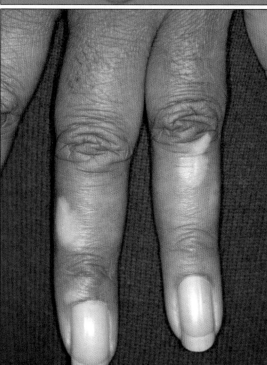

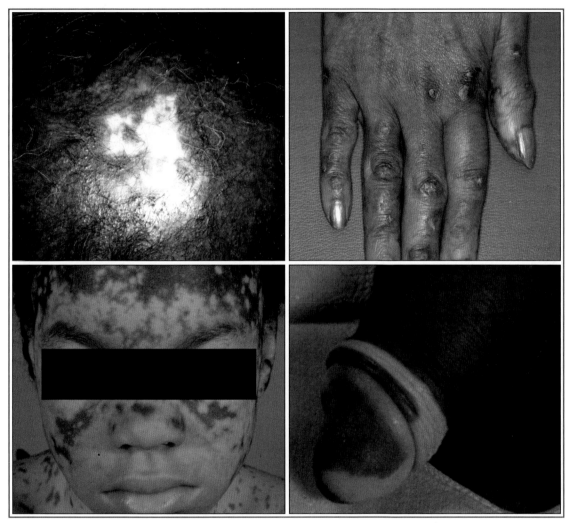

DEFINITION: Vitiligo manifests as symmetrical depigmented patches often beginning on the hands or periorificial regions.

ETIOLOGY: An autoimmune etiology has been proposed since associations with hyperthyroidism, diabetes, alopecia areata and pernicious anemia have been described. Thirty percent of vitiligo patients have a positive family history. Occurrences are usually seen during the first two decades of life.

VITILIGO
(CONTINUED)

CLINICAL PERSPECTIVE: The psychological impact of this disease, especially in darker skinned patients, cannot be exaggerated. Anxiety and the feeling of social stigmatism can accompany the 'white spots' of vitiligo.

Black people may have an unusual trichrome form of Vitiligo. These lesions consist of various hues of depigmentation, hypopigmentation and normal skin. Veloce Vitiligo, a rare occurrence, describes rapid depigmentation over a period of weeks.

DIFFERENTIAL DIAGNOSIS: Discoid lupus erythematosus (follicular plugging, hypopigmentation, often sun-exposed regions); scleroderma (indurated); tinea versicolor (fine scale, truncal location); pityriasis alba (usually malar region, atopic); leprosy (anesthetic, endemic region); piebaldism (white forelock, present at birth), and post-inflammatory hypopigmentation (history of primary dermatosis, trauma, or corticosteroid use) may simulate vitiligo.

TREATMENT OPTIONS: The treatment of Vitiligo often depends on the extent of clinical involvement. If less than 20% of the total body surface (TBS) is affected, topical psoralen and ultraviolet A light (PUVA) is advised. For greater than 20% TBS involvement, oral PUVA is recommended. If 50% or more of the TBS is involved, depigmentation with monobenzone cream is a consideration. Topical corticosteroids may be a viable option in young children who are not candidates for PUVA therapy. Oral pulse corticosteroid therapy has also yielded encouraging results. Surgical modalities including autologous epidermal grafts and melalocyte transplants may prove helpful in certain cases. Innovative treatments for Vitiligo have emerged in recent years. For example, Khellin, a furanochromone, combined with ultraviolet A light (KUVA) may be less phototoxic than PUVA therapy. L-phenylalanine, levamisole, pseudocatalase and calcium have all been employed with varying success.

TABLES

TABLE 1

MEDICATIONS ASSOCIATED WITH PHOTOSENSITIVITY REACTIONS:

PHOTOTOXIC DRUGS

Tetracycline	Isotretinoin
Griseofulvin	Methotrexate
Sulfonamides	5-Fluorouracil
Fluoroquinolones	Ibuprofen
Ketoconazole	Naproxen
Hydrochlorothiazide	Aspirin
Furosemide	

PHOTOALLERGIC DRUGS

Benzodiazepines	Benzocaine
Sulfonamides	Pilocarpine
Piroxicam	Psoralens
Chloroquine	Methyldopa
Nifedipine	Fluorescein dye
Dapsone	

TABLE 2

CAUSES OF LEG ULCERATION

Trauma	External: injuries, burns, scalds, chemical. Self-inflicted: artefacts. Injection ulcers
Infections	
Viral	
Bacterial	Acute: 'desert sore', gas gangrene Chronic: Buruli ulcer, tuberculosis, leprosy, swimming pool granuloma, osteomyelitis
Anaerobic	Meleney's ulcer, synergistic bacterial gangrene (with streptococcus)
Mycotic	Superficial or deep fungus
Spirochetal	Syphilis, yaws
Leishmaniasis	
Infestations and bites	Spiders, scorpions, snakes
Metabolic	Diabetes, gout
Vasculitis	Rheumatoid, systemic lupus, collagen disease, immune complex disease, pyoderma gangrenosum
Perniosis (erythrocyanosis frigida)	

Table 2 continued on next page

TABLES

TABLE 2 (CONTINUED)

CAUSES OF LEG ULCERATION

Venous	Varicose veins
	Congenital absence of veins
	Post-thrombotic
Atrophie blanche	
Necrobiosis lipoidica	
Neoplastic	Epithelioma, Kaposi's sarcoma, leukemia, reticulosis, basal cell carcinoma
Arteriovenous anastomosis	Congenital, traumatic
Ischemic	Scars, fibrosis, radiodermatitis
Arterial	Hypertension (Martorell's), temporal arteritis, atherosclerosis
Thrombosis, embolism, platelet agglutination	
Blood diseases	Polycythemia Spherocytosis, sickle-cell anemia
Skin diseases	Pemphigoid, psoriasis, tinea, summer ulcers
Neuropathic ('trophic')	Diabetes mellitus, leprosy, tabes dorsalis, syringomyelia, neuropathic, decubitus

TABLE 3

DERMATOPHYTES LIKELY TO PREDOMINATE AS CAUSES OF TINEA CAPITIS

M. audouinii	- Nigeria and other parts of West Africa
M. canis	- Colombia, Cuba, Puerto Rico, Argentina, Chile, Uruguay, Venezuela, Denmark, Finland, France, United Kingdom, Spain, South Africa, Saudi Arabia, Australia, New Zealand
M. ferrugineum	- Eastern Europe, Angola, Zaire, Japan, Taiwan
T. tonsurans	- Mexico, Peru, USA
T. violaceum	- Algeria, Egypt, Libya, Tunisia, China, India, West Pakistan
T. schoenleinii	(sporadic only) - Greenland, Morocco, Libya, Iran, Turkey, Iraq, West Pakistan
T. yaoundei	- Cameroons

(Tables 2 and 3 reprinted with kind permission of Rook, Wilkinson, Ebling, Textbook of Dermatology, 5th ed.; Blackwell Scientific Press, Oxford, 1992)

REFERENCES

ACNE KELOIDALIS NUCHAE

1. Halder RM. Hair and scalp disorders in blacks. Cutis 1983, 32: 378-80.
2. Halder RM. Pseudofolliculitis barbae and related disorders. Dermatol Clinics 1988, 6(3): 407-12.
3. Kantor GR, Ratz JL, Wheeland RG. Treatment of acne keloidalis nuchae with carbon dioxide laser. J. Amer Acad Dermatol 1986. 14: 263-7.
4. Kenney JA Jr. Dermatoses common in blacks. Postgrad Med 1977, 61:122.
5. Layton AM, Yip J, Cunliffe WJ. A comparison of intralesional triamcinilone and cryosurgery in the treatment of acne keloids. Br J Dermatol 1994, 130(4): 498-501.
6. Ratzer MA. A clinical trial of flurandrenolone tape. Br J Clin Pract 1970, 24(4): 1-4.
7. Shelly WB, Shelly DE, eds. Advanced Dermatologic Therapy. Philadelphia: W.B. Saunders. 1987: 417-19.

ATOPIC DERMATITIS

8. Arnold HL, Jr. Odom RB, James WD, ed. Atopic dermatitis; eczema; noninfectious immunodeficiency disorders. Andrew's diseases of the skin. Philadelphia: W.B. Saunders, 1990: 68-88.
9. Berger TG, Elias PM; Wintroup BU. Atopic dermatitis, In: Manual of therapy for skin diseases. New York: Churchill Livingstone, 1990: 20-4.
10. Bierman CW, et al. Eczema, rickets and food allergy. J Allergy Clin Immunol 1978, 61: 119.
11. Fergussen DM, et al. Eczema and infant diet. Clin Allergy 1981, 11: 325.
12. Holt LE. The natural history of infantile eczema: Its incidence and course. J Pediatr 1965, 66(part 2): 158.
13. Mathew DJ, et al. Prevention of eczema. Lancet 1977, 1: 321.
14. McLaurin C. Pediatric dermatology in black patients. Dermatol Clinics 1988, 6(3): 45.
15. Molkhou P, Wagnet JC. Food allergy and atopic dermatitis in children: Treatment with Oral sodium cromoglycate. Ann Allergy 1981, 47: 173.
16. Musgrove K. Morgen JK. Infantile eczema. Br J Dermatol 1976, 95: 365.
17. Rosen T. Martin S, ed. Atlas of Black Dermatology. Boston: Little, Brown and Company, 1981: 19-57.
18. Roth HL, Kierland RR. The natural history of atopic dermatitis. Arch Dermatol 1964, 89: 209.
19. Vickers CFH. The natural history of atopic eczema. Acta Derm Venereol (Stockh) 1980, 92 (sup): 113.
20. Vowles M, et al. Infantile eczema. Br J Dermatol 1955, 67: 53.

DERMATOSIS PAPULOSA NIGRA

21. Babapour R, Leach J, Levy H. Dermatosis papulosa nigra in a young child. Pediatric Dermatology 1993, 10(4): 356-8.
22. Grimes PE, Arora S, Minus HR, et al. Dermatosis papulosa nigra. Cutis 1983, 32: 385-6.
23. Hairston MA, Reed RJ, Derbes VJ. Dermatosis papulosa nigra. Arch Dermatol 1964, 89: 655.
24. Kenney JA Jr. Dermatosis papulosa nigra and seborrheic keratosis. Clinical aspects. Ala J Med Sci 1980, 17: 49.
25. Lever WF, Lever GS. Tumors and cysts of the epidermis. In: Histopathology of the skin. Philadelphia: J.B. Lippincott Company. 1990: 523-77.
26. McLaurin Cl. Cutaneous reaction patterns in blacks. Dermatol Clinics 1988, 6(3):353-62.

DISSECTING CELLULITIS OF THE SCALP

27. Adrian RM. Arndt KA. Perifolliculitis capitis: successful control with alternate-day corticosteroids. Ann Plast Surg 1980, 4: 166-9.
28. Baden HP. Diseases of the hair and nails. Chicago: Year book Medical Publishers, 1987: 156-64.
29. Dellon AL, Orlando JC. Perifolliculitis capitis: surgical treatment for the severe cases. Ann Plast Surg 1982, 9: 254-9.
31. Halder RM. Hair and scalp disorders in blacks. Cutis 1983, 32: 378-80.
32. Kligman AM, Mills OH. Acne cosmetica. Arch Dermatol 1957, 75: 509-11.
33. McDonald CJ, Kelly AP. Dermatology and venereology. In: Williams RA, ed. Textbook of black related diseases. New York: McGraw-Hill, 1975: 513-91.
34. McMullen F, Zeligman I. Perifolliculitis capitis abscedens et suffodiens. Its successful treatment with x-ray epilation. Arch Dermatol 1956, 73: 256.
35. Moschella SL, Klein MH Miller RJ. Perifolliculitis capitis abscedens et suffodiens: report of a successful therapeutic scalpings. Arch Dermatol 1967, 96: 195-7.
36. Moyer DG. Perifolliculitis capitis abscedens et suffodiens. Arch Dermatol 1962, 85: 378-84.
37. Ramesh V. Dissecting cellulitis of the scalp in 2 girls. Dermatologica 1990, 180(1): 48-50.
38. Scott DA. Disorders of hair and scalp in blacks. Dermatol Clinics 1988, 6(3): 387-95.
39. Setty LR. Hair patterns of the scalp of white and negro males. Am J Phs Anthropol 1970, 33: 49-55.
40. Shelly WB, Shelly DE, eds. Advanced Dermatologic Therapy. Philadelphia: W.B. Saunders, 1987: 417-19.
41. Williams CN. Dissecting cellulitis of the scalp. Plast Reconst Surg 1986, 77: 378-81.

DRUG INDUCED PHOTOSENSITIVITY REACTION

42. Dahl MV, Photoimmunology. Clinical immunodermatology. St Louis: Mosby 1996, 395-404.
43. Gould JW, Mercurio MG, Elmets CA. Cutaneous photosensitivity diseases induced by exogenous agents. J Amer Acad Dermatol 1995, 33(4): 551-73.
44. Willis I. Photosensitivity reactions in black skin. Dermatol Clinics 1988, 6(3): 369-75.

FOX-FORDYCE DISEASE

45. Effendy I, Ossowski B. Fox-Fordyce disease in a male patient-response to oral retinoid treatment. Clinical and Exper Dermatol 1994, 19(1): 67-9.
46. Fieldman R, Masouye I. Fox-Fordyce disease: successful treatment with topical clindamycin in alcoholic propylene glycol solution. Dermatology 1992, 184(4): 310-13.
47. Giacobetti R, Caro WA, et al. Fox-Fordyce disease: control with tretinoin cream. Arch Dermatol 1979, 115: 1365-66.
48. Graham JH, Shafer JC, et al. Fox-Fordyce disease in male identical twins. Arch Dermatol 1960, 82: 212-21.
49. Helfman RJ. A new treatment for Fox-Fordyce disease. South Med J 1962, 55: 681-84.
50. Kronthal HL, Pomeranz JR, et al. Fox-Fordyce disease. Treatment with an oral contraceptive. Arch Dermatol 1965, 91: 243-5.
51. Lever, WF, Lever GS. Inflammatory diseases of the epidermal appendages and of cartilage. In: Level WF, Lever GS, eds. Histopathology of the skin. Philadelphia: J.B. Lippincott Company, 1990: 218-31.
52. Leyh F. Morbus Fox-Fordyce disease. Uberlegungen zur Pathogenesse. Hautarzt 1973, 24: 482-5.
53. Lottge M, Flache K. Case report of Fox-Fordyce disease. Zentralblatt fur gynakologie 1988, 110(11): 707-9.
54. Pasricha JS, Nayyar KC. Fox-Fordyce disease in the post-menopausal period successfully with electrocoagulation. Dermatologica 1973, 147: 271-274.

55. Pinkus H. Treatment of Fox-Fordyce disease. J. Amer Med Assoc 1973, 223: 924.
56. Rosen T, Martin S. Atlas of Black Dermatology. Boston: Little Brown, 1981; 59-87.
57. Shelley WB. Treatment of Fox-Fordyce disease. J Amer Acad Dermatol 1972, 222: 1069.
58. Storino WD, Engel GH. Office surgical management of recalcitrant axillary lesions. Cutis 1978, 21: 338-41.

FUTCHER'S LINES
59. Brauner GJ. Cutaneous disease in black children. Am J Dis Child 1983, 137: 488-96.
60. Futcher PH. A peculiarity of pigmentation of the upper arm of negroes. Science 1938, 88: 570.
61. Henderson AL. Skin variations in blacks. Cutis 1983, 32: 376-7.
62. James WD, Carter JM, Rodman OG. Pigmentary demarcation lines: a population survey. J Amer Acad Dermatol 1987, 16(3): 584-90.
63. McLaurin CI. Cutaneous reaction patterns in blacks. Dermatol Clinics 1988, 6(3): 353-62.

GINGIVAL HYPERPIGMENTATION
64. Brauner GJ. Cutaneous disease in black children. Amer J Dis Child 1983, 137: 488-96.
65. McLaurin CI. Cutaneous reaction patterns in blacks. Dermatol Clinics 1988, 6(3): 353-62.

IDIOPATHIC GUTTATE HYPOMELANOSIS
66. Blechen SS, Ebling FJG, Champion RH. Disorders of skin colour. In: Rook, Wilkinson, Ebling 5th ed. Textbook of Dermatology. London: Blackwell Scientific Publications 1992: 1561-1622.
67. Cummings KI, Cottel WI. Idiopathic guttate hypomelanosis. Arch Dermatol 1966, 93: 184-6.

KELOIDS
68. Ala-Kokko L, Rintala A, Savolainen ER. Collagen gene expression in keloids: an analysis of collagen metabolism and type 1,2,3,4,5 procollagen mRNAs in keloid tissue and keloid fibroblast cultures. J Invest Dermatol 1987, 89: 238-44.
69. Alster TS. Laser treatment of scars; do lasers really work? Cosmet Dermatol 1995, 8(10): 41-4.
70. Alster TS, Williams CM. Treatment of keloid sternotomy scars with 585 nm flashlamp-pumped pulsed dye laser. Lancet 1995, 345: 1198-2000.
71. Alster TS. Improvement of erythematous and hypertrophic scars by the 585nm flashlamp-pumped pulsed dye laser. Ann Plast Surg 1993, 31: 1-5.
72. Apfelberg DB, Maser MR, White DN, et al. Failure of CO2 laser: excision of keloids. Lasers Surg & Med 1989, 9: 382-8.
73. Berman B, Bieley HC. Adjunct therapies to surgical management of keloids. Dermatol Surg 1996, 22(2): 126-30.
74. Berman B, Bieley HC. Keloids. J Am Acad Dermatol 1995, 33(1): 117-23.
75. Berman B, Duncan MR. Inhibition of dermal fibrosis by interferons. In: Nickoloff BJ, ed. Dermal Immune System. Ann Arbor, MI: CRC Press, Inc., 1993, 209-26.
76. Berman B, Duncan MR. Short-term keloid treatment in vivo with human interferon-alpha 2a results in selective and persistant normalization of keloid fibroblast collagen, glycosaminoglycan and collagenase production in vitro.; J Am Acad Dermatol 1989, 21: 694-706.
77. Bernstein EF, Harisiadis L, Solomon G, et al. Transforming growth factor-beta improves radiation-impaired wounds. J Invest Dermatol 1991, 97(3): 430-4.
78. Border WA, Nobel NA. Transforming growth factor-beta in tissue fibrosis. N Engl J Med 1994, 331: 1286-92.
79. Brenizer AG. Keloid formation in the negro. Ann Surg 1915, 61:87.
80. Carney SA, Cason CG, Gowar JP, et al Cica-Care gel sheeting in the management of hypertrophic scarring. Burns 1994, 20(2): 163-67.
81. Dierickx C, Goldman MP, Fitzpatrick RE. Laser treatment of erythematous/hypertrophic and pigmented scar in 26 patients. Plast Reconstr Surg 1995, 95: 84-90.
82. Escarmant P, Zimmermann S, Amar A, et al. The treatment of 783 keloid scars by iridium 192 interstial irradiation after surgical excision. Int J. Radiat Oncol Biol Phys 1993, 26: 245-51.
83. Fox H. Observations on skin diseases in the american negro. J. Cutan Dis 1908, 26, 67.
84. Fulton JE. Silicone gel sheeting for the prevention and management of evolving hypertrophic and keloid scars. Dermatol Surg 1995, 21(11): 947-51.
85. Gold MA. A controlled clinical trial of topical silicone gel sheeting in the treatment of hypertrophic scars and keloids. J Am Acad Dermatol 1994, 30: 506-7.
86. Goldman MP, Fitzpatrick RE. Laser treatment of scars. Dermatol Surg 1995, 21(8): 685-7.
87. Goslen JB. Wound healing after cosmetic surgery. In: Coleman WP, Hanke CW, Alt TH, Asken TH, Asken S, eds. Cosmetic Surgery in the Skin: Principles and Techniques. Philadelphia: BC Decker, 1991: 47-63.
88. Granstein RD, Rook A, Flotte TJ, et al. A controlled trial of intralesional recombinant interferon-gamma in the treatment of keloidal scarring.
89. Griffith BH, Monroe CW, McKinney P. A follow-up study on the treatment of keloids with triamcinilone acetonide. Plast Reconstr Surg 1970, 46: 145-50.
90. Kantor GR, Wheeland RG, Bailen PL, et al. Treatment of earlobe keloids with carbon dioxide laser excision: a report of 16 cases. J Dermatol Surg Oncol 1985, 11: 1063-7.
91. Katz BE. Silastic (r) gel sheeting found to be effective in scar therapy. Cosmet Dermatol 1992, 5. 32.
92. Katz BE. Silicone gel sheeting in scar therapy. Cutis 1995, 56: 65-7.
93. Kelly AP. Keloids. Dermatol Clinics 1988, 6(3): 412-24.
94. Klumpar DI, Murray JC, Anscher M. Keloids treated with excision followed by radiation therapy. J Am Acad Dermatol 1994, 31: 225-31.
95. Lawrence WT. In search of the optimal treatment of keloids: report of a series and a review of the literature. Ann Plast Surg 1991, 27: 164-78.
96. Lo TC, Seckel BR, Salzman FA, et al. Single-dose electron beam irradiation in treatment and prevention of keloids and hypertrophic scars. Radiother Oncol 1990, 19: 267-72.
97. Mercer NSG. Silicone gel in the treatment of keloid scars. Br J Plast Surg 1989, 42: 82-7.
98. Murray JC. Scars and keloids. Dermatol Clinics 1993, 11(4): 697-708.
99. Multi E. Ponzio E. Cryotherapy in the treatment of keloids. Ann Plast Surg 1983, 3: 227-32.
100. Nemeth AJ. Keloids and hypertrophic scars. J Dermatol. Surg Oncol 1993, 19: 738-46.
101. Norris JCE. The effect of carbon dioxide laser surgery on the recurrence of keloids. Plast Reconstr Surg 1991, 87: 44-9.
102. Olbricht SM, Stern RS, Arndt RA. Co2 laser and cold steel surgical treatment of keloids give comparable results. Lasers Surg Med 1988, 8: 187.
103. Onwukne MF. Surgery and methotrexate for keloids. Schoch Letter 1978, 28:4.
104. Peltonen J, Hsiao LL, Jaakkola S, et al. Activation of collagen gene expression in keloids: co-localization of type I and type VI collagen and transforming growth factor beta 1 mRNA. J Invest Dermatol 1991, 240-7.
105. Pinol G, Rueda F, Marti F, et al. Effect of minoxidil on the DNA synthesis in cultural fibroblasts from healthy skin or keloids. Medicina Cutanea Ibero-Latino-Americana 1990. 18: 13-7.

106. Pollack SV. Management of keloids. In: Wheeland RG, ed Cutaneous Surgery. Philadelphia: W.B. Saunders Company, 1994: 688-98.

107. Priestly GC, Lord R. Stavropoulos P. The metabolism of fibroblasts from normal and fibrotic skin is inhibited by minoxidil in vitro. Br J Dermatol 1991, 125: 217-21.

108. Quinn KJ. Silicone gel in scar treatment. Burns 1987, 13: 33-40.

109. Rusciani L. Use of cryotherapy in the treatment of keloids. J Dermatol Surg Oncol 1993. 19: 529-34.

110. Ship AG, Weiss PR, Mincer FR, et al. Sternal keloids: successful treatment employing surgery and adjunctive radiation. Ann Plast Surg 1993, 31(6): 481-7.

111. Zouboulis CC, Blume U, Buttner P, et al. Outcomes of cryosurgery in keloids and hypertrophic scars. A prospective consecutive trail of case series. Arch Dermatol 1993, 129: 1146-51.

LEUKOEDEMA

112. Duncan SC, Su WPD. Leukoedema of the oral mucosa (possibly an acquired white sponge nevus). Arch Dermatol 1980, 116: 906-8.

113. Van Wyke CW, Ambrosio SC. Leukoedema: Ultrastructural and histochemical observations. J. Oral Pathol 1983, 12: 29-35.

LICHEN NITIDUS

114. Kellett JK, Beck MH. Lichen nitidus associated with distinctive nail changes. Clin Exp Dermatol 1984, 9: 201-4.

115. Kint A, Meysman L, Bugingo G et al. Lichen nitidus and Crohn's disease. Dermatologica 1982, 164: 272-7.

116. McLaurin C. Pediatric dermatology in black patients. Dermatol Clinics 1988, 6(3): 451-73.

117. Natarajan S, Dick DC. Lichen nitidus associated with nail changes. Int J Dermatol 1986, 25: 461-462.

118. Ocampo J, Torne R. Generalized lichen nitidus: report of two cases treated with astemizole. Int J Dermatol 1989, 28: 49-51.

119. Okamoto H, Horio T, Izumi T. Micropapular sarcoidosis simulating lichen nitidus. Dermatologica 1985, 170: 253-55.

120. Randle HW, Sander HM. Treatment of generalized lichen nitidus with PUVA. Int J Dermatol 1986, 25: 330-1.

121. Tanguchi S, Chanoki M, Hamada T. Recurrent generalized lichen nitidus associated with amenorrhea. Acta Dermato-Venereolgica 1994, 74(3): 224-5.

122. Thio HB. Lichen nitidus treated with astemizole. Br J Dermatol 1993, 129: 342.

123. Wilson HTH, Bett DCG. Miliary lesions in lichen planus. Arch Dermatol 1961, 83: 920-3.

124. Wright S. Successful treatment of lichen nitidus. Arch Dermatol 1984, 120: 155-6.

LICHEN PLANUS

125. Bagan JV. Treatment of lichen planus with griseofulvin: Report of seven cases. Oral Surg Oral Med Oral Pathol 1985, 60: 608.

126. Bollag W, Ott F. Treatment of lichen planus with temarotene. Lancet 1989, 2: 974.

127. Higgens EM, et al. Cyclosporin A in the treatment of lichen planus. Arch Dermatol 1989, 125: 1436.

128. Ho VC, et al Treatment of severe lichen planus with cyclosporine. J Am Acad Dermatol 1990, 22: 64

129. Massa MC, Rogers RS III. Griseofulvin therapy in lichen planus. Acta Derm Venerol (Stockh) 1981, 61: 547.

130. McLaurin Cl. Unusual patterns of common dermatoses in blacks. Cutis 1983, 352-60.

131. Ortonne JP, et al. Oral photochemotherapy in the treatment of lichen planus. Clinical results, histopathology and ultrastructural observations. Br J Dermatol 1978, 99: 77.

132. Paslin DA. Sustained remission of generalized lichen planus induced by cyclophosphamide. Arch Dermatol 1985, 121: 236.

133. Rosen T, Martin S, ed. Atlas of Black Dermatology. Boston: Little Brown and Company, 1981: 1-18.

134. Rosen T, Martin S, ed. Atlas of Black Dermatology. Boston: Little, Brown and Company, 1981: 19-57.

135. Sehgal VN, et al. Histopathological evaluation of griseofulvin therapy in lichen planus: A double-blind control study. Dermatologica 1980, 161: 22.

MIDLINE HYPOPIGMENTATION

136. Brauner GJ. Cutaneous disease in black children. Am J Dis Child 1983, 137: 488-96.

137. McLaurin Cl. Cutaneous reaction patterns in blacks. Dermatol Clinics 1988, 6(3): 353-62.

138. Rosen T, Martin S, ed. Atlas of Black Dermatology. Boston: Little, Brown and Company, 1981: 1-18.

139. Seimanowitz V, Krivo JM. Hypopigmented markings in negroes. Int J Dermatol 1973, 12: 229.

140. Weary PE, Behlen CH. Unusual familiar hypopigmentary anomaly. Arch Dermatol 1965, 92: 54.

MONGOLIAN SPOT

141. Gawkrodger DJ. Racial influences on skin disease. In: Rook AJ, Wilkinson DS, Ebling FJG, et al, 5th ed. Textbook of Dermatology. London: Blackwell Scientific Publications, 1992: 2859-75.

142. Hasegawa Y, Yasuhara M. Phakomatosis pigmentovascularis type IVa. Arch Dermatol 1985, 121: 651-55.

143. Osburn K. Schosser RH, Everett MA. Congenital pigmented and vascular lesions in newborn infants. J Amer Acad Dermatol 1987, 16: 788-92.

144. Rosen T, Martin S. Atlas of Black Dermatology, Boston: Little Brown 1981, 59-87.

NAIL PIGMENTATION

145. Leyden JJ, Spott DA, Goldshmidt H. Diffuse and banded melanin pigmentation of nails. Arch Derm 1972, 105: 548-50.

146. Mcnash S. Normal pigmentation of the nails of the negro. Arch Dermatol Syph 1931, 25: 876.

147. Shelley WB, Rawnsley H, Pillsbury D. Postirradiation melanonychia. Arch Dermatol 1964, 90: 174.

NEVUS OF OTA

148. Geronemus RG. Q-switched ruby laser therapy of nevus of Ota. Arch Dermatol 1992, 128(12): 16181-22.

149. Kopf AW, Weiodman Al. Nevus of Ota. Arch Dermatol 1962, 85: 195-208.

150. Liesegang TJ. Pigmented conjunctival and scleral lesions. Mayo Clinic Proceedings 1994, 69/2): 151-61.

151. Liu JC, Ball SF. Nevus of Ota with glaucoma; report of three cases. Ann of Opthamol 1991, 23(8): 286-9.

152. Lowe NJ, Weider JM, Sawcer D, et al. Nevus of Ota: treatment with high energy fluences of the Q-switched ruby laser. J Amer Acad Dermatol 1993, 29(6): 997-1001.

153. Lynn A, Brozena SJ, Espinoza CG, et al. Nevus of Ota aquisata of late onset. Cutis 1993, 51(3): 194-6.

154. Osburn K. Schosser RH Everett MA. Congenital pigmented and vascular lesions in newborn infants. J Amer Acad Dermatol 1987, 16: 788-92.

155. Rosen T, Martin S. Atlas of Black Dermatology. Boston: Little Brown 1981, 59-87.

156. Theunissen P, Spincemaille G, Pannebakker M, et al. Meningeal melanoma associated with Nevus of Ota: case report and review. Clinical Neuropath 1993, 12(3): 125-9.

PALMOPLANTAR HYPERPIGMENTATION

157. Henderson AL. Skin variations in blacks. Cutis 1983, 32: 376-77.
158. McLaurin Cl. Cutaneous reaction patterns in blacks. Dermatol Clinics 1988, 6(3): 352-62.

PITYRIASIS ALBA

159. Bassaly M, Miale A. Studies on pityriasis alba. Arch Dermatol 1963. 88: 272-3.
160. Burton JL. Eczema, lichenification, prurigo and erythroderma. In: Rook AJ, Wilkenson DS, Ebling FJG, et al, 5th ed. Textbook of dermatology. London: Blackwell Scientific Publications, 1992, 537-88.
161. Mosher DB, Fitzpatrick TB, Hori Y, et al: Disorders of melanocytes. In: Fitzpatrick TB, Eisen AZ, Woolf K, et al, eds. Dermatology in general medicine. New York: McGraw-Hill, 1993: 903-5.
162. Urano-Suehisa S, Tagami H. Functional and morphological analysis of the horny layer of pityriasis alba. Acta Derm Venerol (Stockh) 1985, 65: 164-7.
163. Wolf R, Sandbank M. Extensive pityriasis alba and atopic dermatitis. Br J Dermatol 1985, 112: 247.
164. Zaynoun ST, Aftimos BG. Extensive pityriasis alba: a historical histochemical and ultrastructural study. Br J Dermatol 1983, 108: 83-90.
165. Zaynoun ST. Jaber LA. Oral methoxsalen photochemotherapy of extensive pityriasis alba: preliminary report. J Am Acad Dermatol 1986, 15(1): 61-5.

PITYRIASIS ROSEA

166. Andersson CR. Dapsone treatment in a case of vesicular pityriasis rosea. Lancet 1971, 2: 493.
167. Arndt KA, et al. Treatment of pityriasis rosea with UV radiation. Arch Dermatol 1983, 119: 381.
168. Bjornberg A. Epidermal-dermal inflammatory conditions of unknown etiology. In: Fitzpatrick TB, Eisen AZ, Woolf K, et al, eds. Dermatology in general medicine. New York, N.Y.: McGraw-Hill 1993: 1117-23.
169. Chuang TY, Ilstrup DM, Perry HO, et al. Pityriasis rosea in Rochester, Minnesota. 1969-1978. J Am Acad Dermatol 1982, 7: 80-9.
170. Hendricks AA, Lohr JA. Pityriasis in infancy. Arch Dermatol 1979, 115: 896-7.
171. Leonforte JF. Pityriasis rosea: exacerbation with corticosteroid treatment. Dermatologica 1981, 163: 480.
172. McLaurin Cl. Cutaneous reaction patterns in blacks. Dermatol Clinics 1988, 6(3): 352-3.
173. McLaurin Cl. Unusual patterns of common dermatoses in blacks. Cutis 1983, 352-60.
174. Rosen T, Martin S, ed. Atlas of Black Dermatology. Boston: Little, Brown and Company, 1981: 19-57.
175. McPherson A, et al. Is pityriasis rosea an infectious disease? Lancet 1980, 2: 1077.
176. Parsons JM. Pityriasis rosea update: 1986. J Am Acad Dermatol 1986, 15: 159.
177. Vollum DI. Pityriasis rosea in the African. Trans St Johns Hosp Dermatol Soci 1973, 59: 269.

POMADE ACNE

178. Bulengo-Ransby SM. Topical tretinoin therapy for hyperpigmented lesions caused by inflammation of skin in black patients. N Eng J Med 1993, 328: 1438-43.
179. Johnson B. Requirements in cosmetics for black skin. Dermatol Clinics 1988, 6(3): 489-96.
180. Kligman AM, Mills OH. Acne cosmetica. Arch Dermatol 1972, 106: 843-50.

POST-INFLAMMATORY HYPERPIGMENTATION & HYPOPIGMENTATION

181. Breathnach AC, Nazzaro-Porro M, Passi S, et al. Azelaic acid therapy in disorders of pigmentation. Clinics in Dermatology 1989, 7(2): 106-18.
182. McLaurin Cl. Cutaneous reaction patterns in blacks. Dermatol Clinics 1988. 6(3): 352-62.
183. Nguyen QH. Bui TP. Azelaic acid: pharmacokinetic and pharmacodynamic properties and its therapeutic role in hyperpigmentary disorders and acne. Int J Dermatol 1995. 34(2): 75-83.

PSEUDOFOLLICULITIS BARBAE

184. Alexander AM. Evaluation of foil-guarded shaver in the management of pseudo-folliculitis barbae.: Cutis 1981, 27: 534-42.
185. Bouman FG. Surgical depilation for treatment of pseudofolliculitis or local hirsutism of the face. Plast Reconst Surg 1978, 62: 390-5.
186. Brown LA. Pathogenesis and treatment of pseudofolliculitis barbae. Cutis 1983, 32: 373-5.
187. Conte MS, Lawrence JE. Pseudofolliculitis barbae: no "pseudoproblem". J Amer Med Assoc 1979, 241: 53-4.
188. De La Guardia M. Facial depilatories on black skin. Cosmet Toilet 1976, 91: 37-8.
189. Hage JJ, Bouman FG. Surgical depilation for the treatment of pseuydofolliculitis or local hirsutism of the face: experience in first 40 patients. Plast Reconst Surg 1991, 88(3): 446-51.
190. Halder RM. Pseudofolliculitis barbae and related disorders. Dermatol Clinics 1988, 6(3): 407-12.
191. Hall JC, Goetz CS. Pseudofolliculitis-revised concepts of diagnosis and treatment. Report of three cases in women. Cutis 1979, 23: 798-800.
192. Kligman AM, Mills OH Jr. Pseudofolliculitis of the beard and topically applied tretinoin. Arch Dermatol 1973, 107: 551-2.
193. Perricone NV. Treatment of pseudofolliculitis barbae with topical glycolic acid: a report of two studies. Cutis 1993, 62(4): 232-5.
194. Rosen T, Martin S, ed. Atlas of Black Dermatology. Boston: Little, Brown and Company 1981, 89-118.
195. Shelly WB, Shelly DE, eds. Advanced Dermatologic Therapy. Philadelphia: W.B. Saunders, 1987: 417-19.
196. Smith JD, Odome RB. Pseudodfolliculitis capitis. Arch Dermatol 1977, 113: 328-9.

PSORIASIS VULGARIS

197. Frey L. An atlas of psoriasis. Park Ridge, NJ: The Parthenon Publishing Group, Inc. 1992: 1-111.
198. McLaurin Cl, Pediatric dermatology in black patients. Dermatol Clinics 1988, 6(3): 451-73.

SARCOIDOSIS

199. Abeles H, Robins AB, Chaves AD. Sarcoidosis in New York City. Am Rev Resp Dis. 1961, 84: 120-21.
200. Caruthers B, Day TB, Minus HR. Sarcoidosis. A comparison of cutaneous manifestations with chest radiographic changes. J Natl Med Assoc 1975, 67: 364.
201. Cohen HV, Annular Sarcoidosis. Arch Dermatol 1977, 113: 1451.
202. Griffiths CE, Leonard JN, Walker MM. Acquired ichthyosis and sarcoidosis. Clin Exp Dermatol 1986, 11: 361-64.
203. Irgang S. Ulceration of cutaneous lesions in sarcoidosis. Br J. Dermatol 1955, 67-255.
204. James DG, Neville E. Worldwide review of sarcoidosis. Ann NY Acad Sci 1976, 278: 321.
205. Kauh YC, Goody HE, Luscombe HE, Icthyosiform sarcoidosis. Arch Dermatol 1978, 114: 100.

206. Labow TA, Atwood WG, Nelson CT. Sarcoidosis in the american negro. Arch Dermatol 1964, 89-682.
207. Meyers M, Barsky S. Ulcerative sarcoidosis. Arch Dermatol 1978, 114: 447.
208. Minus HR, Grimes PE. Cutaneous manifestations of sarcoidosis in blacks. Cutis 1983, 32: 361-64.
209. Rosen T, Martin S, ed. Atlas of Black Dermatology. Boston: Little, Brown and Company, 1981: 19-57.
210. Sharma OP. Cutaneous sarcoidosis. Clinical features and management. Chest 1972, 61: 320.
211. Sones M, Israel H. Course and prognosis of sarcoidosis. Am J Med 1960, 29: 84.

SEBORRHEIC DERMATITIS

212. Burton JL, Eczema, lichenification, prurigo and erythroderma. In: Rook, Wilkinson, Ebling, 5th ed.; Textbook of Dermatology. London: Blackwell Scientific Publications, 1992: 545-52.
213. McLaurin Cl. Pediatric dermatology in black patients. Dermatol Clinics 1988, 6(3): 457-73.
214. Seghal VN, Saxena AK, Kumari S. Tinea Capitis: a clinicoetiologic correlation. Int J Dermatol 1985, 24: 116-19.
215. Stratigos JD, Antoniou C, Katsambas A, et al. Ketoconazole 2% cream versus Hydrocortisone cream in the treatment of seborrheic dermatitis. J Amer Dermatol 1988, 19: 850-3.

SICKLE CELL LEG ULCERS

216. Al-Momen AK. Recombinant human erythropoietin induced rapid healing of a chronic leg ulcer in a patient with sickle cell disease. Acta Hematologica 1991, 86(1): 46-8.
217. Ankra-Badu GA. Sickle cell leg ulcers in Ghana. East African Med J 1992, 69(7): 366-9.
218. Baum KF, MacFarlane DE. Cupidore L, et al. Corynebacterium diptheriae in sickle cell leg ulcers in Jamaica. West Indian Med J 1985, 34: 24-8.
219. Billett HH, Patel Y, Rivers SP. Venous insufficiency is not the cause of leg ulcers in sickle cell disease. Amer J. Hematol 1991, 37(2): 133-4.
220. Khouri RK, Upton J. Bilateral lower limb salvage with free flaps in a patient with sickle cell ulcers. Ann Plast Surg 1991, 27(6): 574-6.
221. La Grenade L, Thomas PW, Serjeant GR. A randomized controlled trial of solcoseryl and duoderm in chronic sickle cell ulcers. West Indian Med J 1993, 42(3); 121-3.
222. MacFarlane DE, Baum KF, Serjeant GR. Bacteriology of sickle cell ulcers. Trans R Soc Trop Med Hyg 1986, 80: 553-6.
223. Morgan AG. Sickle cell leg ulcers. Int J Dermatol 1985, 24: 643-44.
224. Morgan AG. Proteinuria and leg ulcers in homozygous sickle cell disease, J Trop Med Hyg 1982, 85: 205-8.
225. Rodgers GP, Schechter AN. Noguchi CT, et al. Periodic microcirculatory flow in patients with sickle cell disease. N Eng J Med 1984, 311: 1534-8.
226. Rosen T, Martin S, ed. Atlas of Black Dermatology. Boston: Little, Brown and Company 1981, 89-118.
227. Sehgal SC, Arunkumar BK. Microbial flora and its significance in pathology of sickle cell disease leg ulcers. Infection 1992, 20(2): 86-8.
228. Wethers DL, Ramirez GM, Koshy M, et al. Accelerated healing of chronic sickle cell leg ulcers treated with RGD peptide matrix. Blood 1994, 84(6): 1775-9.

SYPHILIS

229. Berger TG, Elias PM, Wintroup BU. Manual of therapy for skin diseases. New York, N.Y. Churchill Livingstone, 1990. 288-92.
230. Brauner GJ. Cutaneous diseases in blacks. In: Moschella SL, Hurly HJ. Dermatology. Philadelphia: W.B. Saunders, 1985: 1904-45.
231. Buntin DM. Sexually transmitted diseases in blacks. Dermatol Clinics 1988, 6(3): 443-56.
232. Caruthers B. Sarcoidosis. J Natl Med Assoc 1975, 67: 364.
233. Jones J. Bad blood: The Tuskegee syphilis experiment - a tragedy of race and medicine. New York, N.Y.: Free Press, 1981.
234. Rosen T, Martin S, ed. Atlas of Black Dermatology. Boston: Little, Brown and Company, 1981: 19-57.

TINEA CAPITIS

235. Elewski BE, Mercurio MG, DeBenedette V. Recalcitrant tinea capitis may be due to underdosing. Cosmetic Dermatology 1996, 9(2): 57-8.
236. Hay RJ, Roberts SOB, Mackenzie DWR. Mycology. In: Rook, Wilkinson, Ebling, 5th ed.; Textbook of Dermatology. London: Blackwell Scientific Publications, 1992: 1561-1622.
237. Kpea NT, McDonald CJ. Cutaneous infections in blacks. Dermatol Clinics 1988, 6(3): 475-88.
238. Prevost E. The rise and fall of fluorescent tinea capitis. Pediatric Dermatol 1983, 1: 127.
239. Rudolph A. The clinical recognition of tinea capitis from Trichophyton tonsurans. J Amer Med Assoc 1979, 242: 1770.

TINEA VERSICOLOR

240. Arnold HL, Jr., Odom RB, James WD, ed. Diseases due to fungi and yeasts. Andrew's diseases of the skin. Philadelphia: W.B. Saunders, 1990: 318-74.
241. Bamford JTM. Treatment of tinea versicolor with sulfur-salicylic shampoo. J Amer Acad Dermatol 1983, 8: 211.
242. Berger TG, Elias PM, Wintroup BU. Manual of therapy for skin diseases. New York: Churchill Livingstone, 1990: 303-5.
243. Borelli D. Treatment of pityriasis versicolor with ketoconazole. Rev Infect Dis 1980, 2: 592.
244. Faergemann J. Fredericksson T. Propylene glycol in the treatment of tinea versicolor. Acta Derm Venereol (Stockh) 1980, 60: 92.
245. Rosen T, Martin S, ed. Atlas of Black Dermatology. Boston: Little, Brown and Company, 1981: 19-57.
246. Urcuyo FG, Zaias N. The successful treatment of pityriasis versicolor by systemic ketoconazole. J Amer Acad Dermatol 1982, 6: 24.

TRACTION ALOPECIA

247. Costa OG, Junqueira MA. Traumatic alopecia due to traction on hair: comparative study of alopecia luminaris frontalis of Saboraud. Arch Dermatol Syphilo 1943, 48: 5272-32.
248. Earlest RM. Surgical correction of traumatic alopecia marginalis or traction alopecia in black woman. J Dermatol Surg Oncol 1986, 12: 78-82.
249. Halder RM. Hair and scalp disorders in blacks. Cutis 1983, 32: 378-80.
250. Hjorth N. Traumatic marginal alopecia: a special type alopecia Greenlandica. Br J Dermatol 1957, 69: 319-22.
251. Holder WR, Duncan WC. The broken ponytail. Arch Dermatol 1971, 103: 101-2.
252. Lipnik MJ. Traumatic alopecia from brush rollers. Arch Dermatol 1961, 84: 493-5.
253. Rosen T, Martin S. Atlas of Black Dermatology. Boston: Little Brown, 1981: 59-87.
254. Scott DA. Disorders of hair and scalp in blacks. Dermatol Clinics 1988, 6(3): 387-95.
255. Spencer GA. Alopecia luminaris frontalis. Arch Dermatol Syphiol 1941, 44: 1082-85.

VITILIGO

256. Abdel-Fattah A, Aboul-Enein MN, Wassel GM, et al. An approach to the treatment of vitiligo by khellin. Dermatologica 1982, 165: 136-40.

257. Antoniou C, Katsambas A. Guidelines for the treatment of vitiligo., Drugs 1992, 43(4): 490-8.

258. Antoniou C, Schulpis H, Michas T, et al. Vitiligo therapy with oral and topical phenylalanine with UVA exposure. Pharmacol Ther 1989, 545: 28.

259. Ar-Aboosi MM, Ajam ZA. Oral photochemotherapy in vitiligo: follow-up patient compliance. Internat J Dermatol 1995, 34(3): 206-8.

260. Betterle C, Caretto A, DeZio A, et al: Incidence and significance of organ-specific autoimmune disorders in patients with vitiligo. Dermatologica 1985, 171: 419.

261. Brysk MM, Newton RM, Rajaraman S, et al. Repigmentation of vitiliginous skin by cultured cells. Pigment Cell Res 1989, 2: 202-7.

262. Cormane RH, Siddiqui AH, Westerhoff W, et al. Phenylalanine and UVA light for the treatment of vitiligo. Arch of Dermatol Res 1985, 277: 126-30.

263. Cowan CL, Halder RM, Grimes PE, et al. Ocular disturbances in vitiligo. J Am Acad Dermatol 1986, 15: 17.

264. Cunliffe WJ, Hall R, Newell DJ, et al. Vitiligo, thyroid disease and autoimmunity. Br J Dermatol 1968, 80: 135-39.

265. Dawber RPR. Vitiligo in mature onset diabetes. Br J Dermatol 1969, 81: 83-88.

266. Demis J, Weiner MA. Alopecia universalis, onychodystrophy and total vitiligo. Arch Dermatol 1963, 88: 131.

267. El-Mofty AM, El-Sawalhy H, El-Mofty M. Clinical study of a new preparation of 8-methoxpsoralen in photochemotherapy. Int J Dermatol 1994, 33(8): 588-92.

268. Falabella R. Repigmentation of segmental vitiligo by autologous minigrafting. J Am Acad 1988, 9: 514-21.

269. Falabella R. Treatment of localized vitiligo by autologous minigrafting. Arch of Dermatol 1988, 124: 1649-55.

270. Fitzpatrick TB, Elsen AZ, Wolff K, et al. Dermatology in general medicine. New York McGraw-Hill, 1987: 810.

271. Grimes PE. Disorders of hyperpigmentation and hypopigmentation. In Sams M., Lynch P (eds): Principles and practice of dermatology. New York: Churchill Livingstone, 1992: 821-33.

272. Grimes PE. Vitiligo. An overview of therapeutic approaches. Dermatol Clinics 1993, 11(2): 325-38.

273. Grimes PE, Kelly AP, et al. Management of vitiligo in children. Pediatr Dermatol 1987, 3: 498-500.

274. Grimes PE, Kenney JA Jr. Should vitiligo be treated? Cutis 1983, 32: 343.

275. Grimes PE, Minus HR, Chakrabarti SG, et al. Determination of optimal topical photochemotherapy for vitiligo. J Am Acad Dermatol 1982, 7: 771.

276. Halder RM, Pham HN, Breadon JY, Johnson BA. Micropigmentation for the treatment of vitiligo. J Dermato Surg Oncol 1989, 15: 1092-98.

277. Hann SK, Cho MY, Im S, et al. Treatment of vitiligo with oral 5-methoxpsoralen. J Dermatol 1991, 18(6): 324-9.

278. Hann SK, IM S, Bong HW, et al. Treatment of stable vitiligo with autologous epidermal grafting and PUVA. J Am Acad Dermatol 1995, 32(6): 943-8.

279. Hann SK, Kim HI, Im S, et al. The change of melanocyte cytotoxicity after systemic steroid treatment in vitiligo patients. J Dermatol Science 1993, 6(3): 201-5.

280. Hovitz J, Schwartz M. Vitiligo, achlorhydria and pernicious anemia. Lancet 1971, 1: 1331-34.

281. Kao CH, Yu HS. Comparison of the effect of 8-methoxypsoralen (8-MOP) plus UVA (PUVA) on human melanocytes in vitiligo vulgaris and in vitro. J Inv Dermatol 1992, 98(5): 734-40.

282. Kenney JA. Vitiligo. Dermatol Clinics 1988, 6(3): 425-33.

283. Kenney JA Jr.; Vitiligo treatment by psoralens. A long-term follow up study of the permanency of repigmentation. Arch of Dermatol 1971, 103: 475.

284. Kenney JA Jr, Grimes PE: How we treat vitiligo. Cutis 1983, 32: 347.

285. Koga M. Epidermal grafting using the tops of suction blisters in the treatment of vitiligo. Arch Dermatol 1988, 124: 1656-58.

286. Kuiters GR, Middelkamp HV, Siddiqui AH, et al. Oral phenylalanine loading and sunlight as source of UVA radiation in vitiligo on the Caribbean island of Curacao NA. J Trop Med Hyg 1986, 89: 149-55.

287. Kumari J. Vitiligo treated with topical clobetasol propionate. Arch Dermatol 1984, 120: 631.

288. Lerner AB. Repopulation of pigment cells in patients with vitiligo. Arch of Dermatol 1988, 124: 1701-2.

289. Lerner AB, Halaban R, Klaus SN, et al. Transplantation of human melanocytes. J Invest Dermatol 1987, 89: 219-24.

290. Lerner AB, Nordlund JJ. Vitiligo. What is it? Is it important? J Am Med Assoc 1978, 239: 1183-87.

291. Lever WF, Lever GS. Pigmentary disorders. In: Lever WF, Lever GS, eds. Histopathology of the skin. Philadelphia: J.B. Lippincott Company, 1990: 488-93.

292. Nordlund JJ, Halder RM, Grimes P. Management of vitiligo. Dermatol Therapy 1993, 11(1): 27-33.

293. Nordlund JJ, Lerner AB. Vitiligo. Is it important? (editorial) Arch Dermatol 1982, 118: 5-8.

294. Olsson MJ, Juhlin L. Transplantation of melanocytes in vitiligo. Br J Dermatol 1995, 132(4): 587-91.

295. Orecchia G, Perfetti L. Photochemotherapy with topical khellin and sunlight in vitiligo. Dermatol 1992, 184(2): 120-3.

296. Ortel B, Tanew A. Honigsmann H. Treatment of vitiligo with khellin and ultraviolet A. J Am Acad Dermatol 1988, 18: 693-701.

297. Pasricha JS, Khaitan BK. Oral mini-pulse therapy with betamethasone in vitiligo patients having extensive or fast-spreading disease. Int J Dermatol 1993, 32 (10): 753-7.

298. Pasricha JS, Khera V. Effect of prolonged treatment with levamisole on vitiligo with limited and slow-spreading disease. Int J Dermatol 1994, 33(8): 584-87.

299. Plott RT, Brysk MM, Newton R, et al. A surgical treatment of vitiligo. Transplantation of autologous cultured epithelial grafts. J Dermatol Surg Oncol 1989, 15: 1161-66.

300. Skouge JW, Morison WL, Diwan RV, et al. Autografting and PUVA. A combination therapy for vitiligo. Dermatol Surg Oncol 1992. 18(5): 357-60.

301. Siddiqui AH, Stolk LM, Bhaggoe R, et al. L-phenylalanine and UVA irradiation in the treatment of vitiligo. Dermatol 1994, 188(3): 215-8.

302. Wildfang IL, Jacobsen FK, Thestrup-Pederson K. PUVA treatment of vitiligo: a retrospective study of 59 patients. Acta Dermato-Venereologica 1992, 72(4): 305-6.

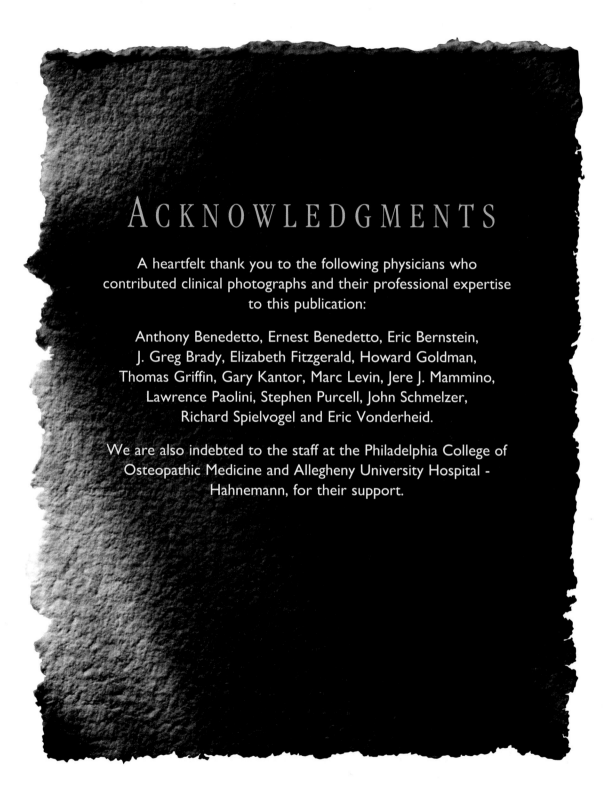

ACKNOWLEDGMENTS

A heartfelt thank you to the following physicians who contributed clinical photographs and their professional expertise to this publication:

Anthony Benedetto, Ernest Benedetto, Eric Bernstein, J. Greg Brady, Elizabeth Fitzgerald, Howard Goldman, Thomas Griffin, Gary Kantor, Marc Levin, Jere J. Mammino, Lawrence Paolini, Stephen Purcell, John Schmelzer, Richard Spielvogel and Eric Vonderheid.

We are also indebted to the staff at the Philadelphia College of Osteopathic Medicine and Allegheny University Hospital - Hahnemann, for their support.

merit
PUBLISHING
INTERNATIONAL